INFORMATION POLLUTION AS SOCIAL HARM

EMERALD STUDIES IN DIGITAL CRIME, TECHNOLOGY AND SOCIAL HARMS

Series Editors: James Martin, Swinburne University of Technology, Australia
Asher Flynn, School of Social Sciences, Monash University, Australia

Previous Volumes:

Cryptomarkets: A Research Companion; James Martin, Jack Cunliffe, Rasmus Munksgaard

The Emerald International Handbook of Technology-Facilitated Violence and Abuse; Jane Bailey, Asher Flynn, Nicola Henry

Over the past two decades, digital technologies have come to permeate ever more aspects of contemporary life. This trend looks to continue and has profound implications for the social sciences, particularly criminology, with technology-facilitated offences now arguably constituting the most dynamic and rapidly growing area of contemporary crime. Despite this development, the discipline of criminology has been slow to embrace the critical study of technology-facilitated offences and social harms, with most research conducted in this area still informed by a relatively narrow range of cybersecurity and applied criminological perspectives.

Emerald Studies in Digital Crime, Technology and Social Harms is part of a new movement within criminology and related disciplines to broaden this narrow focus and engage critically with new trends in technology-facilitated offending and victimisation. The book series uses a combination of critical criminological, socio-legal, and sociological perspectives to consider a wide range of technology-facilitated offences and harmful social practices, ranging from digital surveillance, cyberbullying and image-based sexual abuse through to global darknet drug trading.

EDITORIAL BOARD

Asia Pacific

Professor Mark Andrejevic, Monash University, Australia

Professor Rod Broadhurst, Australian National University, Australia

Dr Akane Kanai, Monash University, Australia

Dr Monique Mann, Queensland University of Technology, Australia

Dr Brady Robards, Monash University, Australia

Dr Campbell Wilson, Monash University, Australia

Europe

Professor Ross Coomber, University of Liverpool, UK

Dr Rutger Leukfeldt, Netherlands Institute for the Study of Crime and Law Enforcement, Netherlands

Dr Adrian Scott, Goldsmiths, University of London, UK

Professor Majid Yar, Lancaster University, UK

North America

Associate Professor Michael Adorjan, University of Calgary, Canada

Professor Walter DeKeseredy, West Virginia University, USA

Professor Benoît Dupont, University of Montreal, Canada

Associate Professor David Maimon, Georgia State University, USA

Assistant Professor James Popham, Wilfrid Laurier University, Canada

INFORMATION POLLUTION AS SOCIAL HARM

Investigating the Digital Drift of Medical Misinformation in a Time of Crisis

ANITA LAVORGNA
University of Southampton, UK

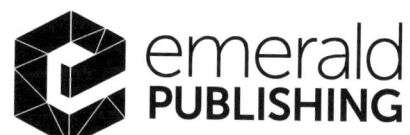

United Kingdom – North America – Japan – India
Malaysia – China

Emerald Publishing Limited
Howard House, Wagon Lane, Bingley BD16 1WA, UK

First edition 2021

© 2021 Emerald Publishing Limited

Reprints and permissions service
Contact: permissions@emeraldinsight.com

No part of this book may be reproduced, stored in a retrieval system, transmitted in any form or by any means electronic, mechanical, photocopying, recording or otherwise without either the prior written permission of the publisher or a licence permitting restricted copying issued in the UK by The Copyright Licensing Agency and in the USA by The Copyright Clearance Center. No responsibility is accepted for the accuracy of information contained in the text, illustrations or advertisements. The opinions expressed in these chapters are not necessarily those of the Author or the publisher.

British Library Cataloguing in Publication Data
A catalogue record for this book is available from the British Library

ISBN: 978-1-80071-522-6 (Print)
ISBN: 978-1-80071-521-9 (Online)
ISBN: 978-1-80071-523-3 (Epub)

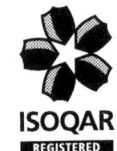

ISOQAR certified
Management System,
awarded to Emerald
for adherence to
Environmental
standard
ISO 14001:2004.

Certificate Number 1985
ISO 14001

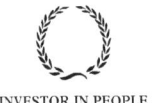

INVESTOR IN PEOPLE

To G. and L., for being the best company I could wish for in this strange year.

"*Our new device of doubt delighted the great public, which snatched the telescope from our hands and turned it on its tormentors*"
—Bertolt Brecht, *Life of Galileo*

CONTENTS

List of Figures — xi
Acknowledgments — xiii

1. Social Harms in Pandemic Times — 1
   1.1. Introduction — 1
   1.2. The Pollution of Medical Information — 3
   1.3. Why Looking at Social Harms? — 8

2. Methodological and Theoretical Approaches — 15
   2.1. Introduction — 15
   2.2. Background of this Book and Notes on Research Methods — 17
   2.3. Drifting into Medical Misinformation: An Integrated Approach — 22

3. Web of Ties: The Actors Behind Medical Misinformation — 27
   3.1. Introduction — 27
   3.2. Receivers — 28
   3.3. Supporters — 30
   3.4. Providers — 34
   3.5. Conspiratorial Ideation and Epistemic Mistrust — 38

4. Building Identities and Networks Through Converging Frames — 43
   4.1. Introduction — 43
   4.2. Narratives of the Self — 44
   4.3. Agency and Empowerment — 53

5. Drifting Off the Polluted Pathway — 57
   5.1. Contexts of Crossdisciplinarity — 57
   5.2. Juggling Divergent Needs — 59
   5.3. Recognizing the Maze — 61

References — 69
Index — 89

LIST OF FIGURES

Fig. 3.1	Drifting into Misinformation	28
Fig. 4.1	Meme on Inverted "Covidiots"	47
Fig. 4.2	Bad Scientists	48
Fig. 4.3	They are Infecting Us	52

ACKNOWLEDGMENTS

A special thanks to AIRIcerca (the Association of Italian Researchers in the world), *AIRInforma* (its science popularization journal), and *Il Post* among the Italian online daily newspapers for helping me stay the course when trying to navigate a sea of polluted information.

1

SOCIAL HARMS IN PANDEMIC TIMES

1.1. INTRODUCTION

In early 2020, the world found itself facing a new challenge, with the outbreak of a novel coronavirus disease – COVID-19, as it was first identified in December 2019 in the Hubei province of China – spreading across countries, to the point that the outbreak was recognized as a pandemic by the World Health Organization (WHO) on March 11, 2020. The virus can cause, among other things, a severe acute respiratory syndrome. The mortality rate directly linked to this virus is estimated to be relatively low, but the impact on public health during the pandemic is considered extremely serious, with some people suffering long term consequences, and because of the progressive breakdown of many healthcare systems due to the number of patients likely to require critical care.

In Italy, the country at the core of the study reported in this book, the virus was first confirmed to be present on January 31, 2020; up to this date, national media reported news of the so-called (at that time) "Chinese coronavirus," and the possibility of facing a pandemic was not part of public debates. In February, with a sharp increase in contagions and deaths, first only some municipalities in northern Italy and then the Lombardia region and whole provinces were placed under quarantine. During the second and third weeks of March, through a series of decrees, the quarantine was extended throughout the country, further limitations restricting the movement of people were imposed, and nearly all commercial activities except for essential businesses and industries were prohibited. In these first stages, the Italian case has been important in framing public health discussions in other countries and, especially in Europe, highlighting a number of concerns around the speed of the virus and potential issues with hospitalization and intensive care if services become overstretched in certain localities (Brown, 2020). Over the Summer, when the situation eased in the country, many restrictions were lifted, and then reinstated, depending on the progression of local outbreaks. At the time of writing, the situation is still very dynamic: after a "second wave" in Autumn and fears of a new rise in numbers linked to the Winter holidays and a new virus variant, new restrictions and (partial) lockdowns in Italy, as well as in other European countries, are starting, are still under development, or are threatened.

The "coronavirus pandemic" struck the world in a very distinctive way: experience from past pandemics or from more recent outbreaks could give us only a limited understanding of how the situation was likely to unfold, as this was the first time that a health crisis – an actual *krisis*, considering how the pandemic led to an unstable and uncertain situation, affecting individuals, communities, and many societies alike (Shaluf et al., 2003) – of this proportion occurred in a world extremely integrated, grounding to a halt economic activities in both wealthy nations and in major emerging market economies and with the fear of a dreadful impact on more vulnerable countries. Social distancing (or, to be more precise, physical distancing) was suggested or imposed in many places as a fundamental factor to mitigate the pandemic and slow its spread – an approach leading to major changes in behavioral patterns and routines of many, as well as impacting mental health and wellbeing.

It is not hard to imagine how this (at least temporary) socio-economic revolution had major effects as regards crime and deviance, challenging criminologists and, more in general, social scientist to study and interpret an evolving context, offering some guidance to "learn" from it and possibly to mitigate some of its most negative outcomes. In this scenario, it is of the upmost importance not only to better conceptualize certain forms of crime (in line with Pemberton, 2007) but also to broaden and deepen criminological knowledge by challenging the very restricted view of "what crime is" to shift attention to other forms of behaviors capable to impact negatively both individuals and society at large. These behaviors might otherwise be overlooked because they are not always and unambiguously against the law. At times, they are not even against social norms, and therefore they might not even be "deviant" by definition. Nonetheless, they might be inherently "bad" (*mala in se*), or lead to a potentially bad outcome.

This book wants to shed light on some of these social practices, and specifically on those that we can group under the umbrella term of health-related "information pollution" (Wardle and Derakhshan, 2017). More in detail, we will look at online medical misinformation and germane practices, conceptualizing them in the broader context of technology-facilitated social harms, with a specific focus on the narratives and conversations taking place in self-identifying alternative lifestyle and counterinformation Italian-speaking online communities.

The remaining part of this first, introductory chapter will provide a more complete presentation of the main concepts and ideas behind this book – that is, *what* are information pollution and medical misinformation, and the added value of using a social harm approach to investigate them through criminological lenses.

1.2. THE POLLUTION OF MEDICAL INFORMATION

In the unfolding of the pandemic, a flurry of (at times conflicting) information has been published and widely disseminated, building up a pile of relevant knowledge alongside equivocal or deceiving news, with the potential of increasing confusion and anxiety – to the point that the term "infodemic" started to be used consistently since mid-February 2020 (Adhanom Ghebreyesus, 2020; Zarocostas, 2020). The infodemic narrative, however, is not sufficiently precise to describe the heterogeneous nature of the information disseminated and shared online, and it can become problematic as it compares the spread of "bad" (or simply confusing, or excessive) information in the current mediascape as a virulent, uncontrolled contagion. As we will see, receivers of information do not simply have a passive role as infected objects of an external agent: in contemporary times and especially in and through cyberspace many receivers are a productive audience, and some even become co-producers of information (Aupers 2020; Stano, 2020).

For these reasons, I prefer to use in this book the notion of *information pollution*, a broader umbrella term that encompasses misinformation (when false information is shared, but no harm is meant), dis-information (when false information is knowingly shared to cause harm), and mal-information (when genuine information is shared to cause harm) (Wardle and Derakhshan, 2017). In proposing this terminology, Wardle and Derakhshan (2017) were detaching themselves from the "fake news" narrative, noticing that it was inadequate to describe the complexity of information misuse (for political purposes, in the cases addressed originally by these authors): in a narrower sense, indeed, "fake news" describes only those news that are verifiably false and that purposely try to mislead their audience. Consistently with the health-related cases of polluted information that we will encounter, also in political misinformation the malicious intent is difficult, if not impossible, to prove, or might genuinely be missing; nonetheless, the consequences can be very problematic.

As anticipated, the phenomenon of information pollution started to receive attention as a distinguishing feature of political life in cyberspace, and more specifically as a variant of information warfare, with the manipulation of information used to obtain a competitive advantage over an adversary. From this perspective, information pollution is nothing new in historical terms. However, the scale of it and its potential impact is revolutionary, as nowadays polluted information can be propagated via countless platforms (Szafranski, 1995; Wall, 2007; Wardle and Derakhshan, 2017), which makes contemporary information pollution particularly subtle and difficult to eradicate (Lavorgna, 2020). Overall, this body of research reported that, among other things, polluted information makes people less knowledgeable, sharpens existing socio-cultural divisions, makes people more skeptical toward legitimate news producers, and also reduces the incentives to invest in accurate reporting (Allcott and Gentzkow, 2017).

Health-related information pollution is a comparable phenomenon that, conversely, has not been addressed yet as a unitary phenomenon; however, there are several studies stemming from medicine, health psychology, health sociology, criminology, and more recently also data science that are useful to provide some background to this work. The subset of fraudulent medical and therapeutic practices has received increasing attention by debunkers and activists over the years, even if only mixed attention in academia: we know that these phenomena are not new, and that despite the consensus in the medical discipline that certain approaches lack scientific evidence, have no biological plausibility or may even be dangerous, the promotion and selling of fake cures and wellbeing approaches advertised as safe and effective has long plagued healthcare systems, often preying on those more vulnerable (Lerner, 1984; Herbert, 1986; Offit, 2013). These practices, however, have boomed in recent years: cyberspace and social media in particular have played a fundamental role in the creation of like-minded virtual networks and in the rise of false experts or fraudulent health specialists exploiting the (badly placed) trust of those looking for hope or for an alternative, easier way to solve their problems (Lavorgna and Di Ronco, 2017; Rojek, 2017; Broniatowski et al., 2018; Klawitter and Hargittai, 2018; Lavorgna and Sugiura, 2019).

In a recent book (Lavorgna and Di Ronco, 2019), these practices – often described as pseudoscience (D'Amato, 2019), quackeries (Lerner, 1984), Complementary and Alternative Medicine (CAM)-adjacent health scams (Lavorgna and Bishop, 2019) or simply frauds (Konnikova, 2016) – were more broadly described as *non-science-based* (or *alternative*) *medical misinformation*. This possibly byzantine label was used with the intent to avoid potentially judgmental designations while being able to comprise a variety of health-related approaches or treatments that were developed in disregard of, or not in full compliance with, scientific standards of modern medicine (Cloatre, 2019). Some of these practices might be seriously dangerous and harmful to people, or carried out with malicious intent, but others may be relatively effectless, have a placebo effect, or simply stem from socio-cultural and epistemological contexts quite removed from western societies.

To understand health-related information pollution and its subset of non-science-based medical misinformation, we need to put them into the broader context of some important changes in medicine occurring in late modernity, as well as in the individual patient–doctor relationship. Trust in medicine has been challenged from two strands: on the one side, the legitimacy of the medical community and its collective expertise has been questioned by some by advancing doubts on the legitimacy of the medical science on which modern medicine depends; on the other side, the individual trust that should be proper of each doctor–patient relationship has been made more complex by the increasing corporatization of medicine (Baron and Berinsky, 2019).

The commercialization of the internet has also profoundly changed health services, with cyberspace being increasingly used to support decision making and to market health products. Alongside opening the way to fascinating developments in healthcare improvements, these changes have the potential for dangerous exploitations. From the one side, patients can now connect more easily among themselves, and with medical practitioners, for instance, with the establishment of self-help communities that have a great potential to provide important information and emotional support, as well as to give patients a sense of empowerment (Ferguson, 1997; Chung, 2014; Fullwood et al., 2019; Zhu et al., 2020). More in general, communication around illness changed especially with and through social media, being transformed from a largely private experience to (at times) a semipublic one (Conrad et al., 2016). On the other side, information accessed via "Dr Google" can be used to self-diagnose a medical condition, to get information on the pros and cons of potential treatments (in a sort of peer-to-peer healthcare, as described by Mackey and Liang, 2017), and even to buy medical products.

Taken together, these aspects are at the basis of the use of the internet as a vector to disseminate medical misinformation and, in some cases, even to carry out frauds, giving individuals a platform to peddle dubious remedies and forms of self-help as better or "alternative" ways of healing than the knowledge and practice of medical expert (Rojek, 2017; Lavorgna and Sugiura, 2019). Through social media networks, questionable messages are easily spread. This form of information pollution can be very difficult to counter, especially because problematic messages distributed via social media are often accessed through the mediation of a friend, a relative, or more generally someone we trust; furthermore, health-related messages broadly distributed via social media tend to contain a mixture of accurate and spurious and unverified information, and hence they look plausible.

In this context, the case that has undoubtedly received most research attention in recent year is the vaccinations one and the rise of the so-called antivax movement, leading to a general decline in global vaccination rates in the last few years, and outbreaks of controllable diseases such as measles and mumps in several countries (Poland and Jacobson, 2011; Hotez, 2019; Ratzan et al., 2019). Indeed, especially in wealthier countries where access to important vaccines is not problematic, rising clusters of unvaccinated people have been linked to the spread of antivaccine misinformation suggesting that vaccinations, especially during early childhood, can cause severe reactions and even conditions such as autism. These unfounded safety concerns, boosted by the well-known Wakefield's scientific fraud (Godlee, 2011), have gained traction over the past few years, especially due to worried parents, fake experts, and cynical public figures trying to please their audiences (Lavorgna and Di Ronco, 2019; Siani, 2019).

In very recent years, a number of studies grounded in data science are playing a prominent role in shedding light on behavioral and communicative patterns in cyberspace. Some have looked at the online diatribe surrounding vaccinations and especially the social networks characterizing antivax online communication, confirming the polarized nature of these debates (Di Ronco and Allen-Robertson, 2019) and suggesting – among other things – that, even if antivax clusters tend to have a smaller average cluster size, they overall provide a larger number of sites for engagement than the pro-vaccination population, hence offering a variety of narratives covering topics such as safety concerns, conspiracy theories, and alternative medicine, being able to attract the interest of a diverse population of individuals (Johnson et al., 2020). Furthermore, antivax clusters are heavily entangled with clusters of undecided individuals, while the pro-vaccination users, being more "isolated," might end up getting the wrong impression that they are dominating the discussion (Johnson et al., 2020).

Data and computer sciences are also increasingly used in efforts to intervene on the "offer" side of polluted information, for instance, trying to use filtering software to improve automatization in detecting mis- and dis-information, or to develop better technologies for automatically detecting fake accounts and bots spreading it, and for deprioritizing updates from sources consistently posting clickbait headlines. On the one hand, the solutions offered by these approaches, while important, are not yet satisfactory – and in fact systems currently employed by social media companies are still very ineffective. On the one hand, technological sophistication makes these tasks more difficult by the day, creating a sort of vicious circle of technological arm race (O'Connor and Weatherall, 2019). It should be kept in mind that not only individuals naively pollute information moved by political or ideological motivations, but there are also polluter information enterprises moved by profit (as viral news create traffic toward certain websites drawing advertising revenue) and major political actors involved, which can resort to very sophisticated *modus operandi*. Moreover, the encrypted nature of many online conversations – which is a plus for other forms of security – makes misinformation extremely difficult to police or somehow moderate. On the contrary, these big data-driven approaches tend to neglect socio-cultural factors in their methodologies of choice: for instance, both traditional filtering (based, for instance, on keywords) and natural language processing do not work well with mis- or polluted information, as what can be considered "mis-" or "polluted" is influenced by cultural and discursive contexts – in a way that closely resembles the issues in using filtering approaches in detecting hate speech, when software for the automatic recognition cannot understand the nuances of certain content, with the consequence that the human intervention is still irreplaceable (Schmidt and Wiegand, 2017; Lavorgna, 2020).

Unfortunately, also existing regulatory frameworks are not very fit for purpose to address information pollution, even if at the moment of writing there are increased attempts (pushed by regulatory institutions, and more or less reluctantly accepted by social media companies and other online intermediaries, which still tend to downplay the influence of their platforms) to intervene to counter and mitigate the effects of at least the more serious forms of dis- and misinformation, in the effort to make our societies more resilient toward cyberharms (Donovan, 2020; Lavorgna, 2020).

It would be of the upmost importance to intervene also on the "demand" side of information pollution but this is an equally daunting task. Indeed, among the reasons behind the success of polluted information are the facts that it is cheap to obtain, difficult to identify, and enjoyable: it is more pleasant for consumers to read a partisan news in line with their system of beliefs, rather than something questioning them (Allcott and Gentzkow, 2017), and – reportedly – social media can easily function as echo chambers where all participants are ideologically aligned. Furthermore, many people might not have the cultural instruments to distinguish what is "polluted" from what is not, and in any case the whole issue touches upon the very delicate equilibria needed to promote and protect the right to freedom of opinion and expression.

While this work focuses on social media, before concluding this section it is important to stress that also traditional media (such as printed or online newspapers and television news) have a big deal of responsibility in promoting, and spreading, polluted information. Even if social media have increasingly become a relevant source of information, traditional forms of media are still the most popular way for people to access news (when combining them with newspaper websites and apps), with the exception of post-Millennials (Gentilviso and Aikat, 2019; Kennedy and Prat, 2019). As such, traditional media still have a major societal role in shaping our perceptions of what is a "problem" and in influencing the solutions that are taken to counter it. Previous research on media representation of medical misinformation showed how printed news (including in Italy), for instance, over time failed to report important issues related to risk and safety of alternative medicine (Weeks and Strudsholm, 2008), and failed to provide a useful distinction between harmful and non-harmful (or even fraudulent) treatments, as they never fully recognized the negative implications brought about by them (Lavorgna and Di Ronco, 2018; Lavorgna and Bishop, 2019). The very same issues were easily observed during the pandemic in Italian newspapers, and it is at least very likely that the confusion generated by many news outlet – especially in their coverage of scientific information – had an impact toward the general public, for instance, influencing the willingness to oblige to protective behaviors (such as wearing masks and maintaining physical distancing). This issue, of course, has not affected only Italy; in many countries official information sources were perceived as untrustworthy, setting the climate for a perfect storm for polluted information, with potential life-saving information (at times emerging information, in a context where it was difficult to clearly identify meaningful information in a clear-cut way) being lost in a tornado of rumors, doubts, and unfounded speculations. This resulted in a very complicated landscape, which showed clearly that the challenge to be met goes beyond debunking a piece of bad information; rather, this has to do with trust, fear, and dissent (Larson, 2020).

1.3. WHY LOOKING AT SOCIAL HARMS?

With very few exceptions (see Section 2.2), criminologists have mostly overlooked (potentially) dangerous non-science-based health practices as a topic of investigation, both as regards some unquestionably illegal practices (see, for instance, the health frauds discussed in Lavorgna and Di Ronco, 2017) and, more in general, the potentially negative impact of these practices on vulnerable individuals even when they do not clearly meet the legal threshold. Nonetheless these practices, and more broadly health-related information pollution and its subset of medical misinformation, should deserve a full-fledged place within the wide constellation of criminological imagination – or at least, I will argue, they are perfect candidates to be considered through the social harm lenses.

Criminology, and the emerging so-called cybercriminology even more, tends to focus on a relatively limited range of core topics, often with a positivistic focus especially in the Anglo-sphere (Powell et al., 2018; Lavorgna, 2020). In this context, the criticisms of those lamenting the degree to which mainstream criminology seems to ask questions and address the issues demanded by the crime control industry (Pemberton, 2007) are of particular relevance. Indeed, a critical approach to criminology – at the cost, maybe, to "stretch" the discipline a little – can have the merit to shed light on forms of crime and deviance that might otherwise be overlooked even if capable of causing great suffering. This holds true particularly in cyberspace, as the seriousness of many harms that are facilitated by digital means, but which are very tangible and real for their victims, tends to be underestimated (Powell and Henry, 2017; Lavorgna, 2021a).

"Harm" is a broad concept that can be associated to emotional or material negativity (Muncie, 2000) or to the non-fulfillment of individuals' needs (Pemberton, 2016). It has been categorized into physical harm, financial or economic harm, emotional or psychological harm, and cultural safety harm (Hillyard and Tombs, 2008; see also Agrafiotis et al., 2016, 2018 for a similar taxonomy of cyberharms). Harms can be suffered by the primary victim (who experiences the act or omission), but also by secondary victims (who suffer financially or emotionally from the harm, even if they are not directly affected by the act or omission), and even tertiary victims (those who experience the harm only vicariously, for instance, when victimization extends to the societal level) (Virtanen, 2017; Lavorgna, 2020). Harms can be caused by both action and inaction, and as stressed by Pemberton (2004, 2007) harms can be caused not only by people's intention but also by indifference, which is "morally comparable" to intent when the person had the chance to change the course of events that led to the production of harm by intervening (Pemberton, 2007) – an effective way to broaden up the coverage of responsibility.

There are a number of reasons as to why looking at "harms" might be preferable to looking at "crimes" in the context of health-related information pollution. First of all, such an approach allows us to bring our understanding and conceptualization of relevant behaviors beyond state definitions of crime (Hillyard et al., 2004), an approach that is particularly promising when investigating events and activities that often occur in "gray" areas of legality, or that can take place at a cross-border level. Furthermore, cyberspace is a socio-legal context evolving extremely fast not only because of technological innovations, but also because of the changes taking place in the political and economic arenas of our "information age" – changes with important legal and ethical implications, on a time when legal frameworks and social perceptions on cyberthreats and risks are yet to be settled (Boyle, 1996; Lavorgna, 2021a).

Second, by looking at "harms" we can avoid the misalignment between criminal law and harmful (or potentially harmful) antisocial behaviors. Discourses on "crime," on the one hand, evoke a certain level of seriousness, hence giving legitimacy to the expansion of the crime control industry, even in front of relatively minor events. On the other hand, the same term "crime" excludes serious behaviors that, especially on an individual level, are nothing more than "micro-deviations" (Popham, 2018), sometimes because culpability might be almost impossible to prove, and sometimes because certain acts are only marginal to the dominant policy (and consequently law enforcement and academic) agendas (Hillyard and Tombs, 2008). This misalignment between criminal law and antisocial behaviors is particularly evident in cyberspace (Lavorgna, 2021a): in a context where low-impact acts can lead to large aggregated losses and significant distress (Wall, 2007) and some forms of deviance are becoming normalized, only by surpassing a legalistic approach to crime it becomes possible to improve our understanding of the real impact of crime, deviance, and (otherwise) hidden harms.

Even if the harm principle ("harm to others," Feinberg, 1984) can be a legitimate ground for criminalizing behavior in modern liberal societies (Simester and Von Hirsch, 2011; Peršak, 2007), it is important to stress that in no way this contribution aims to suggest that many, if not most, of the behaviors observed in the following chapters should be criminalized. First, *ad hoc* regulatory intervention would be problematic in a field where the notion of what "health-related misinformation" (or even "fraud," in some cases) is varies in time and space, if only because scientific norms evolve, and health standards are often culture dependent (Urquiza-Haas and Cloatre, 2019). Furthermore, regulatory intervention in a contested area might lead to unintended consequences such as the "forbidden fruit effect" (Grabosky et al., 1998): some internet actors might work to create alternative points of access to the material or services forbidden in an ideological attempt to respond to what is perceived by them as a form of censorship. In theory, for the most extreme of the behaviors encountered there are already laws and regulations in place (such as those addressing frauds, medical negligence, or even some forms of quackeries as in the case of the UK Cancer Act of

1939), even if too often they are not effectively implemented (Lavorgna and Carr, 2021).

Rather, what should become clearer through the continuation of this book is the urgent need to better acknowledge not only the social, but also the criminological relevance of non-criminal yet harmful behaviors, even when this means to move beyond discussions on the allocation of legal responsibility to individuals, and to better reflect on issues of collective, corporate, or even moral responsibility (Hillyard and Tombs, 2008). In a way, indeed, the distinction between criminal and social harms parallels the one between criminal and moral responsibility: moral agents might not be legally responsible for an act or omission, but they might still (ethically) deserve blame or punishment rather than praise or reward, as a matter of personal or general deterrence (Fischer and Ravizza, 1998; Howard, 2017). This is particularly relevant in a context where, even in cases of full-blown social harms, the criminal harm might not be present because of the lack of *mens rea*, which makes it extremely difficult to prosecute some of these cases through the criminal justice system – an approach that is not always satisfying, as intent can be difficult to prove, and in certain cases indifference could also be culpable (Remain, 1979; Hillyard and Tombs, 2008; Lavorgna, 2021a).

The partial misalignments between criminal law and harmful (or potentially harmful) antisocial behaviors (Hillyard et al., 2004; Hillyard and Tombs, 2008) could be clearly observed in the unfolding of the pandemic, where alongside the emergence (or adaptation) of criminal acts (some of which are likely to receive a lot of academic interest in the coming years, with criminologists already investigating how criminal patterns have been changing/might/will change during the pandemic), we can also observe behaviors leading to potentially serious harms but that tend to be overlooked in traditional criminological discourses.

By observing the unfolding and evolution of the pandemic, it is possible indeed to observe different types of behaviors that can be linked to severe social (and only at times, criminal) harms. While the rest of this book will focus only on one of those – that is, information pollution and its subset of non-science-based medical misinformation – the remaining part of this background section aims to offer a broader contextualization of social behaviors reacting to the novel coronavirus within the social harm literature by stressing how different types of behaviors – some of which are at the fringes of mainstream criminological boundaries – had/are having a role in worsening the social harms suffered in the pandemic and, as such, should receive criminological attention.

First, is the group of those trying outrightly to profiteer from the pandemic. At times, this happened with acts that are already criminalized by the criminal justice system: think, for instance, of the episodes registered in many countries and reported by local and national media of people deliberately coughing to others as a harassing or threatening act that can be prosecuted, for instance, as assault (CPS, 2020). Plenty of examples can be found in the cybercrime arena, with heinous offenders using phishing attacks exploiting worries over COVID-19 to access personal data (NCSC, 2020), or even targeting hospitals with ransomware attacks (*Wired*, 2020). Another area of much interest is the one concerning COVID-19-related frauds. An interesting example is the one reported already in the very early stages of the pandemic (March) by the City of London Police (2020): after a joint investigation by the City of London Police's Intellectual Property Crime Unit, the Medicines and Healthcare products Regulatory Agency, and the United States Food and Drug Administration, a British man was accused of making and selling across the world fake (but potentially dangerous, because of the chemicals used) COVID-19 treatment kits, and charged with one count of fraud by false representation, one count of possession of articles for use in fraud, and one count of unlawfully manufacturing a medicinal product.

Other acts, however, are more difficult to be identified immediately as frauds, and at least for the moment being they might fall more accurately in the "social harms" rather than in the "criminal harms" box. Consider, for instance, the following issue. Vaccine and drug clinical trials are slow to account for safety, as time is needed to monitor both effectiveness and possible side-effects. In a pandemic, however, time is both a matter of public health and money, and in the run against time to tackle the crisis the usual, at time lengthy, procedures to get proper accreditation or certification by the relevant authorities have been eased or waived. Again in mid-March 2020, while researchers from all over the world were still running against time to improve testing kits and serological tests (that is, tests to be used to determine whether a certain individual was infected and has already recovered from the virus) to be distributed in vast scale, it was already possible to find adverts online for rapid, at-home tests produced by some private companies. At that time, however, there was still very little evidence of the accuracy of these early tests, and indeed the hype around their use soon slowed down; but if and when distributed to people not sufficiently informed, they might have led to potentially very dangerous consequences, as both false positive or false negative results might induce individuals to take risky (for themselves, and for others) behaviors.

A second group of interest to stress the relevance of the social harm approach is provided by those who, when it started to become clear that the outbreak was there to last, started hoarding food and household items, as well as disinfectant products, medicines, masks, and gloves. Buying in excess is something generally not receiving criminological attention – rather, it is something encouraged by consumerism – but what when overbuying creates major societal and healthcare problems? It has been reported that panic buying has caused problems in ensuring access to food and essential items to those more vulnerable; at the beginning of the pandemic, for instance, people with lupus have experiences in shortage of vital drugs as they were believed to be effective to treat COVID-19 (The Guardian, 2020a, 2020b; WHO, 2020).

The third group of interest is formed by those who, willingly or moved by ignorance, arrogance, the pursuit of a personal gain and maybe the fear of the economic impact, have downplayed the (potential) impact of the outbreak, promoting a "business as usual" approach while losing precious days or weeks in testing and isolating relevant parts of the populations, or in preparing the healthcare systems with the supplies needed. Such attitude, that has been observed in many countries – among the most notable examples, are the United Kingdom (with the initial British "health exceptionalism" until the U-turn in mid-March leading to a progressive lockdown of the country), Sweden, Brazil, and the United States – was at first present also in Italy – which was ahead of other Western countries in the epidemiological curve. Until early March, indeed, also in Italy the public perception of the outbreak was still polarized, and many of the restriction posed were contested and opposed as "exaggerations." In late February, for instance, the campaigns "Milan does not stop" and "Bergamo is running" were supported by the majors of what soon became among the most severely hit cities (both in Lombardia), and became very popular on social media. In a way, this latter approach can be interpreted as the very unfortunate outcome of cognitive bias (Pisano et al., 2020), or as the materialization of the overreliance of (necessarily superficial, in lack of sufficient scientific evidence) risks assessments at the expense of a proper application of the precautionary principle – that is, the idea that when there is potential serious and irreversible harm and the scientific evidence is inconclusive, the prescribed course of action should be precautionary action – in a public health issue (Pless, 2003; Richter et al., 2005; Vineis, 2005).

In all the cases addressed so far, the social harm approach can help to raise critical awareness on the role and responsibilities of a range of diverse (moral) actors in the context of crime and deviancy during the pandemic. The case of online medical misinformation, a sub-type of information pollution, offers probably the best example. With cyberspace being increasingly used to support health-related decision making and to market health products (Mackey and Liang, 2017), the social implications of online health misinformation are extremely relevant, as they may cause financial, physical, and psychological/emotional harms to the primary victims, as well as public health problems, and loss of confidence in the professional scientific and medical norms (Cattaneo and Corbellini, 2014; Lavorgna, 2021a). As such, our fourth group of interest encompasses the initiators and participants of (self-identifying) alternative lifestyle and counterinformation online communities that, in the context of the pandemic, have proactively used cyberspace, and especially social media, to promote non-science-based medical misinformation and conspiratorial ideas – ranging from boycotting the use of masks and physical distancing, to proactively opposing the use of the COVID-19 candidate vaccines when they become available, to promoting the use of useless or even dangerous substances to prevent or resist the virus. In an overwhelming majority of cases, these behaviors are not illegal; nonetheless, if and when followed, these unfounded advices create a range of negative impacts.

The activities of this fourth group are particularly interesting (yet challenging) to be framed through the harms' lenses, as many of these potentially harmful behaviors seem to originate (at least in some instances, as we will see in Chapter 3) from a genuine spiritual search and the willingness to help and inform others – something noble in principle, but still leading to social harms that should not be overlooked.

2

METHODOLOGICAL AND THEORETICAL APPROACHES

2.1. INTRODUCTION

While the previous introductory chapter set the scope of this book, this second chapter focuses on the *how*, or, in other words, it will present the methodological and theoretical approaches this study relies on. Overall, in a context of increasing "digital positivism" based on big data research methods and computational criminology in online research (approaches that the author herself has used, combined with qualitative analyses, in the context of medical misinformation, see, for instance, Lavorgna and Carr, 2021; Lavorgna et al., 2021), this work wants to stress the importance to retain a space also for qualitative analyses of smaller datasets focusing on interpretative and critical approaches (Fuchs, 2019). Indeed, while recognizing the fundamental importance of recent analyses on polluted information online carried out relying on large amount of data and/or (semi)automated data gathering or analytical processes (among others, Del Vicario et al., 2016; Schmidt et al., 2018; Johnson et al., 2020), in this work I wanted to "zoom in" and look more closely at some of the online social networks that might be identified also through some of these big data approaches, to scrutinize them more in detail: who is involved in these online networks, and who are the individuals behind some "key" social media profiles? What moves them? What makes this type of polluted information so popular, and successful? And, most of all, what makes many people to believe such (mis)information, and to promote it to others?

Through a constructivist epistemology, this study certainly does not aim at identifying ultimate laws, but it rather aims to offer meanings that are relevant through interpretation (Geertz, 1973; Hayward and Young, 2004), challenging the reductionist idea (still very common in the positivistic turn of much cyberspace research) that we need necessarily to quantify and measure human behavior to build our knowledge of it (Lavorgna, 2021b) – the risk, otherwise, is to enter a sort of war against information pollution without having sufficiently understood first important nuances of this phenomenon. Following Hayward and Young's metaphor of the "dual city" (adapted from Raban, 1974 and de Certeau, 1984), while recognizing the importance of studying a city by looking, for instance, at its planning and it demographic, here I aim to look at the same city from a completely different perspective – that is, the experiential city of intersubjectivity and interaction (Hayward, 2004). Positioning myself alongside – and not in opposition – the emerging literature of computational studies on online misinformation, through its different methodological approach this study wants to go below the thinly veil not accessible through positivistic routes. After all, the importance to use both quantitative and qualitative method approaches when dealing with social media data to improve our capacity to make social claims has been already stressed in the literature (see, for instance, Halford et al., 2018).

Theoretically, this study integrates socialization approaches (and specifically the recent adaptation of Matza's ideas with the "digital drift" concept) with cultural approaches. As stressed in the introductory chapter, only a minority of the behaviors encountered in this book can be easily considered as "deviant" (if only because that would imply a sufficient level of societal consensus around science-based approaches or at least around a recognized "value" of science in the society, something that tends to fluctuate depending on many factors such as the topic under discussion, the geographical location, and religious or political identification – see Krause et al., 2019), and only very few of these behaviors are (potentially) illegal. Furthermore, in cyberspace, and especially in certain social media, certain behaviors that would be probably considered (at least borderline) deviant offline suddenly become prevalent among specific populations, making it particularly hard to classify them as "against the norm"; after all, ideas about deviance change over time, and these processes are often boosted and accelerated by new social possibilities provided by technological innovations (Blevins and Holt, 2009). Hence, by relying on a theoretical understanding developed for the study of crime and deviance, there is no implication that the behaviors considered in our study should be criminalized or "upgraded" to a deviancy status. Nonetheless, because of the (potential or actual) harm they can contribute to, theories of deviance can offer precious help in unpacking important behavioral dynamics. We have already discussed how many of the practices observed in this study can create, more or less directly, social harms; it is the normalization and promotion of these practices within certain groups to be problematic. This study aims at better understanding of how this form of problematic socialization takes place and is maintained, looking not only at the individual level (see also Lavorgna and Myles, 2021) but also at the broader cultural ingroup/outgroup (meso)level.

While this chapter focuses on the main socio-criminological approaches embedding this study, the book will also refer to frameworks traditionally belonging to different disciplines, such as anthropology, psychology, and science communication. We will soon see, for instance, how in our everyday handling of uncertainty and risk, a combination of the rational and the magical is not uncommon (Zinn, 2008; Alaszewski, 2015; Brown, 2020). As such, in understanding people's reactions to COVID-19 risks, it is important to look also at people's approaches to precariousness and unpredictability, factors and mechanisms for science denial, and public health communications – something that colleagues from other disciplines have long addressed.

2.2. BACKGROUND OF THIS BOOK AND NOTES ON RESEARCH METHODS

The study reported in this book has been carried out throughout 2020, in the unfolding of the "first" and "second" waves of COVID-19 in Italy (and in many other countries), the lockdowns, and the attempts to return to "normal" pushed mainly by economic considerations, while witnessing the resurgence of several new hotspots, and new closures. This work, however, is also very indebted to some earlier work carried out over the past five years and developed thanks to some small grants of the University of Southampton that gave me the opportunity to start cross-disciplinary dialogues and collaborations with inspiring colleagues through a number of studies (Lavorgna and Di Ronco, 2017, 2018; Lavorgna and Bishop, 2019; Lavorgna and Horsburgh, 2019; Lavorgna and Sugiura, 2019; Lavorgna and Carr, 2021). Additionally, this work has certainly gained from data and insights gathered and developed in the context of two other interdisciplinary analyses carried out over the first half of 2020 (Lavorgna and Myles, 2021; Lavorgna et al., 2021), in the midst of the coronavirus pandemic.

The methodological approach used for this book mainly relies on passive virtual ethnography (Androutsopoulos, 2008; Kozinets, 2010), which was complemented through a small number of narrative interviews with providers and propagators of polluted health-related information.

Ethnography in an immersive type of research that allows an iterative-inductive approach, which evolves and adapts in design as the study progresses, and acknowledges the researcher's own role in this process (Pink et al., 2016): humans, in other words, are recognized as part object and part subject of the study (O'Reilly, 2005). In the context of this research, this approach facilitated treating cyberspace as an environment, experiencing directly from it (Bricken, 1991; Donath, 1996) while observing participants in online conversations and analyzing thematically publicly available material.

When the COVID-19 issue emerged, first in the form of outbreaks and then as a pandemic, I was monitoring already some online (open) Facebook pages and groups in a non-systematic way to follow the latest discussions on alternative medicine and lifestyles, gathering insights for my pre-existing research interest on harmful non-science-based health practices. With the advent of COVID-19, it was impossible to ignore the attention this issue started to receive in those groups, which gave me the possibility to observe the object of this study and its evolution from its outset. After all, it is not unusual for digital ethnographers to witness the rise or major changes of the social worlds they are researching even over a short period of time (Pink et al., 2016). Additionally, in the context of an exploratory psycho-criminological analysis of self-identifying alternative lifestyle online communities – defined as an aggregation of individuals interacting around a shared interest in a way supported and mediated by technology, and guided by some protocols and norms (adapted from Porter, 2004) – during the pandemic (Lavorgna and Myles, 2021), I soon started to monitor very closely one of these Italian-speaking active communities, which was pivoting around a dedicated open Facebook page and a digital magazine. It soon became evident how there was much more to read, and to untangle.

This is why, for this study, I decided from the outset to adopt a more flexible approach compared to the one followed in the above-mentioned study: I did not put any limit to the extent of my online data gathering, with the only pre-determined constraint being the fact that I had to limit myself to information available in "open" spaces for ethical reasons. I also decided to restrict myself at information that was clearly targeted to Italian-speaking users, as this was the linguistic boundary of my study. I monitored data published from January to December 2020, starting from a dozen of Facebook pages, groups, and personal websites I was already aware were discussing health-related information, and following any relevant link suggested or otherwise available, moving from one page to another, from one lead to another, until data saturation was deemed to be reached as no new relevant themes were emerging.

The study was approved by my Faculty Research Ethics Committee (Ethics and Research Governance Online – ERGOII 55870 and 59235.A1).[1]

The digital landscape at the core of this investigation comprises a range of both written text and audiovisual material. I read documents when they were posted, often in forms of screenshots, watched videos, smiled (or not) at memes, followed links to personal websites, forums, and other social media accounts. The pages, groups, and accounts considered range from a few hundred followers up to half million. Most of them had a broad scope, and health-related information was presented and discussed alongside other contemporary topics, ranging from national and international politics to spirituality. However, it soon became clear that all my sources were associated with a specific ethos toward the self, and were somehow interrelated though a shared emphasis on existentialism, transcendence, and personal growth. In total, I looked at more than 200 among social media groups and personal pages, a couple of dozens of websites, and at about 50 videos, audio files, and webinars, which can be estimated in about 750 hours of online observation, spanned across 12 months – something I guess I should partially thank the lockdowns for ….

As agreed by my Faculty Research Ethics Committee, research notes were taken (by hand) on webpages, discussions, images, and videos; a number of posts and images of particular relevance were manually copy-pasted in a Word file for manual analysis, and anonymized at the moment of collection. Considering that the data used for this study were often socially sensitive (as it contained, among other things, political opinions, religious and philosophical beliefs, health information, and potentially information on illegal behaviors), this practical strategy was guided by the effort to minimize ethical risks (particularly as regards the storage of identifying or sensitive information, which were not specifically needed for the scope of this research, and to mitigate the impact of lack of informed consent). Furthermore, this approach was also informed by the need to safeguard the privacy and anonymity of the individuals observed, while ensuring the respect of existing guidelines for online research on social media and the policies of the platform accessed. As mentioned above, the study was limited to information *openly* available online (for instance, I never accessed closed groups on social media), where it could be assumed that the participants expected the virtual space used to be public, in line with current research standards (BSA, 2017; Zimmer and Kinder-Kurlanda, 2017; Social Data Lab, 2019; Lavorgna and Holt, 2021). For concerns related to users' anonymity, personal identifiers are never used in this book, and identifiable quotes have been avoided (Williams et al., 2017); when quotes are used, they have been appropriately modified.

The elements of the ethnographic method used to inform the immersive approach employed in this study have allowed to address health-related information pollution in the context of the pandemic by encompassing relevant contextual understanding (Postill and Pink, 2012; Pink et al., 2016), allowing the capture and analysis of both narratives and conversations of interest in their spontaneity, without having to incite or direct them (Jowett, 2015; Brooker et al., 2017); these naturally occurring interactions reveal internal conventions, mechanisms, and motivations (Goffman, 1983; Sacks, 1992; Giles et al., 2015; Housley et al., 2017). As imagery and picture sharing are an important socio-esthetic parts of online visual conversations, self-presentation, and construction of the digital self, also videos and images (such as memes but also "motivational" pictures) were taken into consideration (McDonald, 2007; Mandoki, 2016). After all, to borrow Katz' words, self-portrayal and storytelling extend beyond linguistic boundaries (Katz, 1988). Narratives (though both written and visual elements) proved to be particularly useful to look at the construction of social identities, being revealing of the perceptions of the self. Some research participants (and specifically some providers and some of the most active supporters, see Section 3.2) even published online, in textual or visual forms, autobiographical accounts allowing to uncover the dynamics of an individual's self-relations and self-understandings (Yar, 2014). By creating, using, and distributing stories, we tell about who we (believe we) are and how we want others to "see" us (Copes and Ragland, 2016; Copes et al., 2019) at the personal level, but we can also create broad social classifications of abstract actors representing generic social types, or develop group identities (Loseke, 2007).

Looking at online narratives and communications suffers the intrinsic limitation of looking (only) at a computer-mediated contacts; also, it allows only to see actors directly engaging in discourses, leaving somehow out from the analysis the silent majority that is simply observing, and likely learning from (Akers, 2009), those online communications. Nonetheless, these type of data have become common in the social sciences over the last two decades, and proved to be a very effective tool to demonstrate relationships between individuals and provide insight into the type of information exchanged between online users (Blevins and Holt, 2009), especially when the nature of the social media considered suggests that individuals have little gain from providing inaccurate or false information. Online sociality, as described by Pink et al. (2016, p. 110), is in fact characterized by a sort of "public intimacy": participants in online conversations on (public) online spaces are aware that potentially everyone might read their words; at the same time, however, as many online threads have a quasi-oral nature, it is recognized that the same participants may feel as they are sharing a conversation within an intimate group of people, and thus can be very open in expressing their thoughts. After all, especially during the harsher stages of the pandemic, online spaces were *the* places where many discussions could occur. Furthermore, in cyberspace users become co-producer of relevant content (Fuchs et al., 2010) also by having an increased ability to choose which contents to share (or not) with their personal networks, hence co-defining what is a newsworthy story, promoting a certain framing, and creating a "viral reality" (Postil, 2014).

My initial plan was to complement my research data with a number of narrative interviews (Schütze, 1983) in order to provide an opportunity to key research participants to narrate their own stories, experiences, and motivation to myself (the researcher-listener). I contacted a total of 32 administrators and moderators of social media groups and pages pivoting around (and disseminating) potentially harmful health-related polluted information. I decided to not contact individuals without a specific "formal" role in the social media observed as I did not want my potential respondents to feel somehow ambushed in what was clearly for them a safe space; also, having anonymized relevant comments at the moment of data collection, it would have been very unpractical to purposely sample the respondents. I also decided to not contact some very notorious and highly visible (but confrontational) individuals openly promoting medical misinformation who enjoy a guru-like status among their very active and at time verbally aggressive followers – as observed during the ethnography. As to comply with ethics I had to present myself with my real name, I wanted to avoid excessive personal exposure to minimize risks of online harassment toward myself and my family.

As we will see in the following chapters, is it not unusual for my potential respondents to have strong, negative opinions toward institutionalized forms of knowledge (including Universities); they tend not to trust anything perceived as imposed, official, or formal – let alone reading lengthy information sheets and signing consent forms. Out of the 32 administrators and moderators contacted, only 11 replied; among those, two did an oral interview, one answered to my questions in writing; others said that they would have been happy to talk but not to sign the consent form, so I had to stop my communications with them. To comply with the requests of the Research Ethics Committee, as my information sheet broadly mentioned "a study on health-related online discussions in the context of COVID-19" (as it would have been impossible to approach the designated respondents presenting the study as research on misinformation), I had to ask my three respondents to sign also a debriefing form at the end. Only one interviewee agreed to sign it. The problems encountered in carrying out the narrative interviews expose some very common issues faced by researchers pursuing direct contacts with potential interviewees during online ethnography on controversial and polarized topics, existing ethics loopholes, and the consequent tensions affecting power dynamics in interviews, and researchers' private and public selves. These issues have been discussed in detail in a recent research note (Lavorgna and Sugiura, 2020).

2.3. DRIFTING INTO MEDICAL MISINFORMATION: AN INTEGRATED APPROACH

Drawing from the interactionist and constructionist notion that identity formation occurs socially, and conformity and deviance are to be located mostly at the micro-level (that is, people interact one with another, defining and redefining values and norms in this process, Thompson and Gibbs, 2017), this study departs from the assumption that there is not a pervasive rigid social structure defining conformity and deviance. As emerged already in the Introduction to this book, medical misinformation is often a fluid concept, where different societal groups may define the same behavior as normal, deviant, to be criminalized, or to be welcomed depending on their varying systems of attitudes and beliefs, or their social networks. In this context, the only macro-level, or systemic, parameter we can probably agree on pivots around the idea of "harm" as something to be prevented or mitigated for the societal and possibly the individual good – and even in this case, an agreement on what "harm" is might be difficult to reach. What might be considered by some an economic harm (for instance, an expensive supplement with no proven health benefit), might be seen by others as a way to enhance individual wellbeing, a way to take self-care, a harmless placebo.

In line with this premise, the approach used in this book builds on recent theoretical developments on technology-enabled offending, and specifically on the conceptual framework of digital drift proposed by Goldsmith and Brewer (2015) and further expanded – among others – by Holt et al. (2019), which extends elements of Matza's original formulation of drift to cyberspace. This approach is here integrated with elements of cultural criminology, which offers a useful framework to encompass how digital drifts occurs within a specific (sub)cultural context, which plays a pivotal role in identity construction. In a way, integrating these approaches offers some useful lenses to look at the interplay between the individual and the meso level, thus helping to unpack at a deeper level the behavioral dynamics facilitating the success of medical misinformation online.

In his sociological etiology of delinquency, Matza (1964, p. 28) used the idea of "drift" to convey a specific image: that of an individual who is "casually, intermittently, and transiently immersed" in patters of illegal or deviant actions, investing in them sufficiently to elicit a sense of satisfaction and even prestige, but not enough to be or become unreceptive to other more conventional patterns and behaviors (to which he or she rather actively participates); the ideological and psychological traits do not preclude neither deviant nor conventional actions. Drift "stands midway between freedom and control," and is "a motion gently guided by underlying influences" (p. 29). In other words, the equilibrium between conformity and wrongdoing is a shifting one, depending on specific situations and circumstances such as exposure to nonconform peers or belief systems (especially when it comes to youth socialization), which allows to neutralize or justify involvement in delinquency. It is here argued that the same dynamics explain the varying degree of active participation in the promotion and propagation of health-related polluted information and misinformation, whose attractiveness depends on an equally varying exposure to networks normalizing and even encouraging antiscientific or otherwise antiofficial ideas and ideologies.

In contrast with subcultural theories, Matza's work rejects the idea of subcultural systems of values and norms, with peer groups setting standards of behavior and normative constraints (Haines, 1981). Matza, conversely, sustains that individuals engaging in delinquency are rarely committed to an alternative set of values, drifting among norms and behaviors as opportune to them and escaping the dominant normative constraints through neutralization (Sykes and Matza, 1957; Matza, 1964). Furthermore, the motivation for much delinquency can be found in values (think of bohemian, or radicalism) that are "subterranean" of conventional society, being recognized and accepted – at least in their mild forms – by many (Matza and Sykes, 1961). Hence, there is no clear dichotomy between convention and deviance, as deviance mostly depends on situational aspects. Also, the perceived lack of legitimacy (due, for instance, to incompetence or inconsistency in action, or by viewing the system actors as flawed and hypocritical) or of effectiveness (because people are not hold accountable for their actions, and there are no real consequences for offending) of the criminal justice system can lead toward delinquency, creating a "sense of injustice" toward authorities: individuals feel freed from social norms, and their behaviors will become dependent once more on situational factors (Matza, 1964, p. 148; Holt et al., 2019).

By adopting a naturalistic perspective, Matza (1969) emphasized the importance to maintain a non-judgmental, empathic attitude of "appreciation" of deviance, which should be looked from the inside; otherwise, we risk to lose the capacity to understand deviants' personal meanings, and hence to understand their acts (Haines, 1981) – an attitude that was upheld throughout this study, enabled by the methodologies of choice. Indeed, Matza (1964, p. 9) explicitly critiqued the hard determinism characterizing positivist approaches in the study of deviancy, favoring a softer determinism that allows to consider both choice and constraint as elements of humanity, recognizing that there is a complex interplay between determination and will: each individual is both free and constrained, depending on the specific context; some are freer than others because of personal qualities and/or social circumstances (Haines, 1981).

Goldsmith and Brewer (2015) furthered these ideas, adapting them to the virtual world. Cyberspace is here interpreted as a set of places, often readably accessible (and leavable) in both synchronous and asynchronous ways, and that allow for social encounters and interactions. The underlying idea is that cyberspace has reconfigured the social arrangements for criminal and deviant acts, impacting on the level of individual commitment to deviant activities and lifestyles by allowing individual actors to limit their involvement in particular groups (as they can more easily "drift" in and out of them), loosening group boundaries while expanding the range of possible interactions. In other words, according to this view, because of the mediated effect of cyberspace on human interactions and personal commitment, deviant identities are not (or less) stable. By focusing especially on young offending, they suggest that the escapism provided by the virtual world and the relative absence of capable guardians exposes individuals to transgressive influences, allowing and even encouraging flirtation with them (Goldsmith and Brewer, 2015; Holt et al., 2019).

The need to look at the "drift" in cybercrime and cyberdeviance, Goldsmith and Brewer (2015) suggest, depends also on the fact that cyberspace is used for leisure and entertainment purposes, and (in an increasingly number of countries) it has a high degree of social penetration, thus challenging our traditional conceptions of criminal and deviant interactions while contributing to the formation of prospective subcultures. Initial exposure to certain groups can often occur incidentally, with individuals not being aware of the existence of a broader social group promoting certain norms and values, whose presence might become clearer only at a later point (Holt et al., 2019).

The "drift" framework, especially in its digital variant, resonated immediately very well with the behaviors I was observing in my research, inspiring me to answer to the invitation (Holt et al., 2019) to further examine its value in improving our understanding of pathways into problematic socialization online, and the role of neutralizing beliefs in transitioning in and out certain systems of beliefs. Of course, as we will see, some adaptations are necessary, if only because of the intrinsic distinction between deviant vs (potentially) harmful behavior, and because I will argue that the notion of subculture does not reflect appropriately the fluid interactions characterizing the creation, propagation, and support of medical misinformation online – rather, we have a constellation of more or less loosely formed collectives drawn together by diverse yet convergent narratives.

Additionally, there is an important aspect touched upon in Goldsmith and Brewer (2015) but it is not fully developed which I think deserves more attention: the role of cyberspace in enabling both individual and ingroup identity construction. Goldsmith and Brewer recognize that the internet enables forms of self-curation and the pursuit of identity-related interests such as hobbies, and that ingroup interactions might strengthen and amplify shared feelings of abuse, or to be victims of an unjust system – but these aspects are only briefly covered to stress the need of further research into the nature of online interactions in an optic of crime prevention and reduction, and to discourage antisocial uses of the internet. In this study, I will expand on these aspects, integrating some element of cultural criminology.

Cultural criminology is about viewing crime as a creative construct or product by placing it in the context of culture – seen as something in constant evolution (Hayward and Young, 2004), closely interconnected with collective meaning and collective identity (Ferrell et al., 2008). It draws from interactionist sociology, cultural studies, and critical theory to investigate, among other things, experiential dynamics of deviant subcultures, the mediated construction of crime and crime control issues, and the relationship between crime, crime control, and cultural spaces (including the media) (Ferrell, 1999). In line with Matza's approach, also cultural criminology departs from a naturalistic stand, embracing the idea of complexity of the human being and human agency, and stressing the need to use qualitative approaches – a "methodology of attentiveness," to borrow Ferrell and Hamm's (1998) words – to identify and interpret the lifestyle(s), the existing rich narrative of symbolism, the esthetic, and the transgression to social norms in a highly reflexive way (Geertz, 1973; Hayward and Young, 2004). Through cultural criminology, emotions and irrationality are included in explanations of crime and deviance.

Furthermore, cultural criminology perspectives are very effective to unpack the politics of crime as emerging through anticrime campaign, through the cultural construction of deviancy and marginality, and through the resistance of certain subcultures to legal control (Young, 1999, p. 398). The idea of transgression (and crime and deviancy as forms of transgression) pays a key role in this framework: the act of transgression has attractiveness in itself, as it is seen as the way to attempt a solution to what is (at least perceived as) a problem, an injustice, or an ontological insecurity (Hayward and Young, 2004). The deeper roots of these dynamics, according to cultural criminologists, are to be found in the features and the constraints of late modernity and the creation of "a bulimic society where massive cultural inclusion is accompanied by systematic structural exclusion" (Young, 2003, p. 397), which have created a fertile ground for individuals to rely on forms of transgression to reassert their identity, finding new ways to seek a form of realization (Young, 2003; Hayward and Young, 2004). In this context, crime's nature becomes "sensual," risk-taking creates a form of pleasure, and hence risk becomes a challenge rather than a deterrent (Young, 2003).

The construction of both personal and group identities through a process of differentiation and the development of an "us vs them" narrative, as we will see, are central to the creation and propagation of medical misinformation, and in the associated risk-taking attitude. The feeling of taking control of information and a renewed sense of agency thus become the instruments that those (who perceive themselves as structurally) excluded have to oppose the system to restore their lost freedoms.

NOTE

1. Note that ERGOII is the name of the University System (it stands for Ethics and Research Governance Online). A number of anonymous reviewers are assigned to each ERGO application.

3

WEB OF TIES: THE ACTORS BEHIND MEDICAL MISINFORMATION

3.1. INTRODUCTION

Expanding on previous work based on both criminological and psychological understanding, this chapter and the next one present the main types of actors behind much medical misinformation, discussing their declared and apparent individual motivations as well as the epistemic and narrative frames at the core of their (online) identity construction. At the basis of these chapters is the idea that, when online, we form impressions of each other, and we all use a range of different signals to establish and promote our online identity or identities (Donath, 1996, 2014). In line with Goffman's (1959, 1963) notion of "regulation," people in social interactions perform like in a play and manage impressions through a careful presentation of themselves, especially when they are trying to appear as "respectable" (Yar, 2014; Sugiura, 2018). Especially providers, but also some supporters and utilizers present themselves by relying on several narratives online and using various storytelling techniques – which can be object of analysis.

This chapter in particular will present the actors encountered in this study by categorizing them as *providers* (those actively involved in offering non-science-based health approaches), *supporters/propagators* (those who proactively support one or more providers, becoming an important source of polluted information), and *receivers/utilizers* (those who belong to a certain online group but mainly as bystanders, or participate in a very limited role; when they support the provider, the support is quite limited, for instance, through occasional "likes"). Of course, a certain degree of overlap exists between these different types of actors: the proposed classification is useful for analytical needs, but it is worth noting that, depending on the circumstances (or the

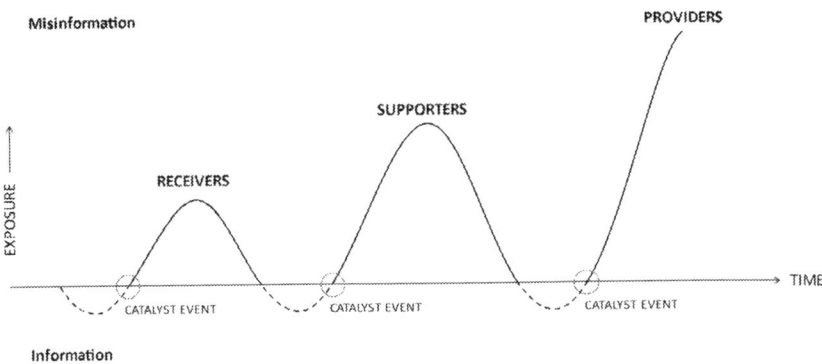

Fig. 3.1. **Drifting into Misinformation.**

platform used), the same actor might fit in a different category. Furthermore, the belonging to a certain category can change overtime: as we will see, many providers used to be supporters, or passive receivers.

If we imagine to place the extent of digital drift along a continuum, these different categories of actors are to be progressively placed in different parts of it; the further they are positioned along the continuum, the more their presence in online health-related discourses shapes their identity (Fig. 3.1). Advancement through the continuum is generally prompted by a catalysis event, that pushes or pulls individuals further, changing the equilibria in the drift. These positions, in other words, reflect different degrees of involvement and attachment associated to their online participation, as some individuals are or become more invested than others (Licoppe and Inada, 2012). As such, these different degrees become indicative of digital drift (Goldsmith and Brewer, 2015).

3.2. RECEIVERS

Receivers of health-related polluted information (and, among them, utilizers of useless or harmful treatments) are the silent majority of this study. If we were to graphically look at our individuals through the lenses of social networks' analyses, we would see them at the very margins of the network, rarely involved in core conversations. When we look at them qualitatively, we see an assortment of very different individuals that, taken together, cannot be seen as part of a clearly identifiable community, and there is no or very little evidence that they display specific subcultural characteristics. These individuals simply cluster in transient and loosely formed collectives around a common interest or activity (Forsyth, 2019), resembling more a crowd of strangers springing up around a specific hashtag, a page, or a thread because they are curious about something that is happening, and want to know more. When we look at the information available in their public profiles, we find a variety of men and women of different age groups and with different educational or professional background; we see the so-called general public; we might even spot some of our friends or acquaintances (as it happened to me, as Facebook's algorithms puts at the very top of those listed as members of a certain group those that are part of your own network) – regardless of the biological implausibility or the conspiracist ideation behind certain notions and approaches, indeed in line with research suggesting that conspiratorial thinking should no longer be considered a feature of fringe beliefs (Goldberg, 2008; Mirable and Horne, 2019; Pierre, 2020).

Receivers' involvement in the propagation of polluted information online is overall limited: for instance, even in social media groups with thousands of followers, problematic posts are rarely liked or shared in the hundreds. Receivers tend to be bystanders. Sometimes, though, they comment below some posts, or engage in limited conversations. From these limited interactions, we learn that they sometime sustain or express admiration for certain providers or certain ideas, at least because they are aligned with their systems of belief (*"this is true, I noticed it as well"*; *"this is precisely what I do think, this is all correct!"*; *"this is a truthful note"*; *"this is one of the most interesting and accurate pages of the Italian internet"*). Other times, however, they are simply looking for specific information (*"could someone give me more detailed information on the video of [name], MD? Is it true that in the flu vaccine there were two coronaviruses?"*; *"Dear [name], I friended you [on Facebook] in the hope you can help my son to get better"*; *"Dear doctor, but should we do the same homeoprophylaxis* [that is, the controversial use of homeopathy as a preventive against serious infectious diseases] *also to our children?"*) – something that might end up putting them in the position of victims of medical misinformation. Utilizers, however, do not recognize their current or potential status as victims; rather, at times, they feel victimized by the State for being denied the "right to try" (new or alternative therapies), and hence for restricting their freedom (*"they are limiting our freedom under the guise of a medical dictatorship"*). In this regard, it is worth stressing that the "no harm in trying" approach can be very tricky to sustain, as the *caveat emptor* ("let the buyer beware") position is very problematic when products or services cause harms (Lerner, 1984).

Apart from gathering health-related information, some receivers are likely to disseminate this information beyond the groups observed in the ethnography, which is worrisome as (physical or virtual) word-of-mouth is an important factor affecting health behavior (Martin, 2017): indeed, there are often requests from within the group to divulge information "outside" among friends and acquaintances to help propagate the ideas presented by providers and supporters within the communities observed. At times, these requests are moved by the urgency that "*they [unspecified people] will soon censor it [a certain material shared in the group].*"

Conventional medical treatments are mentioned, and at times even praised ("*I agree that food is an important component of prevention ad cure, but without conventional medicine and surgery my mum won't be still here today*"; fundraising for a children's hospital was advertised). As suggested by Barcan (2015), the relative peripheral status of certain practices allows them to coexist and even have links with the medical mainstream. So, especially during the "first wave," the efforts of doctors and nurses during the pandemic are generally recognized ("*I deeply respect and thank all those at the forefront of the fight against the new coronavirus, all those working in intensive care*" – even though it should be noted that other users often replied with laughing smileys to this type of sentences). For most people, relying on potentially harmful practices and non-science-based medical approaches is not about ideological rupture or transgression to dominant social norms; as we will see more in detail in the following chapter, for many alternative medical practices simply represent a way to stress personal choices about nature, individualism, and personal responsibility (Martin and Debons, 2015). Also, receivers tend to express doubts rather than certainties ("*I might end up thinking this is all nonsense … but while in doubt I accept this might be true, I can still change my mind*"). Overall, they are looking for something *more*, or *different* – something that they strive for and (reportedly) fail to find elsewhere.

3.3. SUPPORTERS

Supporters play and ambivalent role: on the one hand, they are interested in being active participants in the community they feel part of and try to help or be helped; in some cases, they might even be victims, for instance, in cases of frauds. On the other hand, however, they have the moral responsibility of facilitating the dissemination and adoption of potentially dangerous practices by lending their support to practitioners, also when they have caused proven harms (Lavorgna and Di Ronco, 2017). From this perspective, they can be both victims *and* offenders, which place them in a complex and rare (but not unique, in criminological understanding – see Davies et al., 2017) position in the axis of vulnerability.

Also, in the case of supporters, the group is a heterogeneous one ranging from people with a general interest in alternative medicine or lifestyle having a desire to communicate with like-minded people, to desperate patients (or their beloved ones) trying to get some help or hope, to people aiming to "redeem" or "save" the society, being harshly critical toward governments, the pharmaceutical industry, the medical establishment, and the like (Lavorgna and Di Ronco, 2017). Stressing the co-existence of different types of motivations, at times in apparent conflict with one another, is very important to reject simplistic representations of supporters of non-science-based health practices, which too often tend to be simply depicted as "gullible" (Ernst, 2019; Metin et al., 2020). Among supporters, we find people self-identifying themselves – among other things – as lawyers, life coaches, businessmen/entrepreneurs, philosophers, artists, and independent learners.

Their support role is generally made explicit through their active participation in relevant social media: they create or post relevant material, persistently like and share medical misinformation, and steer conversations (often replying to other users' questions) in the direction of their preferred providers/alternative practices. The most active supporters create content to be uploaded and discussed via social media in an interactive way, as already observed in the case of conspiracy theorists who become simultaneously "prosumers" (Ritzer and Jurgenson, 2010) or "produser" (Bruns, 2008) of content, decoding and encoding information (Aupers, 2020). In some cases, they have groups, pages, and threads specifically dedicated to promoting or advocating for one or more named providers, especially when they feel these providers have been unjustly attacked, mistreated, or discredited; or to make them known to Italian-speaking users, when these providers have been previously active abroad (one supporter, for instance, created a page to promote the upcoming translation of a provider curing "*diseases considered uncurbable by the official medicine*"). In one case, the provider was likely to be a family member (because of the shared family name). Supporters also proactively promote offline events, symposia, and workshops where their favorite providers are going to be present. At times, they give (online and offline) contact details of those health practitioners that they consider valid. Just one example, among many: when I tried to contact one of these supporters (the administrator of a Facebook page promoting a range of COVID-19-related non-science-based treatments while discrediting or mocking preventive measures to counter the spread of the virus) as potential interviewee, I received an automatic reply listing nine different providers with their mobile phone numbers and websites, all presented as "*serious professional practitioners for the health of the body and the spirit. I know them all personally.*"

Supporters were once receivers. When they discuss their personal experiences, we learn that they got interested into unconventional medical (and wellness) approaches generally as (relatively) young adults while "*trying to find [their] true-self*" and often after the encounter with someone who introduced them to a certain life philosophy ("*the call for me arrived when I was 30, and I started to study [a list of alternative health-related practices]; at the same time, the person who was meant to support me in this path entered my life*"), or after some personal disappointment experienced with science-based, westernized medicine ("*I am speaking for personal experience, this* [reportedly not been cured with sufficient care, in the context of the pandemic] *happened to a member of my family*"; "*I have been following you for years, you saved my life*").

As receivers, they were fascinated by alternative practices after an initial (at times, incidental) exposure to (more or less) subterranean networks, starting to drift in and out of them depending on situational aspects (such as gathering information on childhood vaccinations; or the need to "know more" while facing the uncertainties of the pandemic for some of the latest receivers). They became supporters when they got more involved in these networks after the happening of some catalysis event (such as a personal encounter, or some form of personal or professional distress). After the catalysis event, in other words, the commitment of these individuals to certain groups and lifestyles increased, and they became more aware of the existence of broader and readably accessible like-minded social groups promoting convergent (to theirs) norms and values.

In the context of the pandemic, disappointment with the official (governmental, regional, or local) responses was a recurrent key driver, creating – again in line with Matza's framework – a heartfelt sense of lack or legitimacy and effectiveness toward public authorities. As a concerned parent co-founder of a highly frequented Facebook group (at the origin of other Telegram and WhatsApp groups, and of offline manifestations) opposing the use of masks and physical distancing in schools explained: "*During the lockdown we adopted a system that is too rigid, they focused on providing schools with new desks with wheels – it looks like a joke! They cannot guarantee physical distance, it's ridiculous, it's a waste of public money.*" It should be of no surprise that, in the context of a systemically underfunded education sector, the use of public resources for something that is not perceived as a real priority but rather as hygiene theater created a lot of discontent. It is worth noting that, according to the Italian National Institute of Statistics, about 15% of families with a minor do not have computers or tablets, and only a bit more than 20% of families have one device per person, with significant differences between the North and the South of the country (ISTAT, 2020); school building's safety, especially considering the seismic vulnerability of many parts of the country, is still a pressing issue (ImparareSicuri, 2020).

Similarly, inconsistencies in public policies and gross mistakes followed by lack of accountability, such as during the confused and flawed political choices carried out by some municipalities during the first stages of the outbreaks (consider, for instance, the social media campaigns aiming to keep business as usual in hardly hit areas, as discussed in Section 1.3) undermined public confidence (*"they should go to jail"*), making individual behavior more dependent on situational factors.

Also, the perceived lack of legitimacy and effectiveness of the medical and scientific establishment became a catalysis event, making individuals feel freed from following their advices (such as maintaining physical distancing or wearing protective masks, to the point that antimasks hashtags were often used) if not perceived as convenient to them. In the Italian context of the pandemic, "celebrity scientists" (Fahy and Lewenstein, 2014) were harshly attacked and criticized in the fora analyzed, accused of creating additional uncertainties by opposing each other's views in public debates (*"they are doing it only for visibility"*; *"they should spend their time working [in their labs], not fighting for money on tv"*; *"they are not real experts, they are just know-it-all"*). Notable is the example of star virologist Burioni, who become a sort of media celebrity initially by fighting vaccine skeptics (even if he has been criticized by science communicators for his abrasive "blasts" to even mild opponents), and that during the first stages of the pandemic become very popular on television talks and social media, backing up protective measures. In the unfolding of the pandemic, Burioni entered into public forms of disagreement not only with some discredited scientists considered by most part of the scientific community as providers of medical misinformation, but also with other recognized experts (for instance, through a rebuttal via Twitter against the doctor and medical debunker Di Grazia with heated, divisive voices, and a clash with virologist Gismondo as she initially said that the emergency was likely to be over with the Summer). While diverse views are normal in science when approaching a new, evolving phenomenon, this divisiveness was broadly commented and interpreted by supporters as a sign of ineptitude and inadequacy of those informing the "official" public discourse.

In line with the literature on deviant online communities (Maratea and Kavanaugh, 2012), supporters tend to reinforce their identities, and are generally keen to maintain a collegial and sympathetic spirit in the group(s) they are active in, as if it was a safe zone. Negative remarks are directed toward those considered as outsiders, or presenting and defending ideas that are divergent from the spirit of the group. Indeed, supporters seem to feel a strong sense of belonging toward communities aligned with their system of beliefs, and generally are active in shaping, or trying to shape, the identity of the group they feel to belong to – generally showing support to those they see as sufficiently lined up to their views. Support is also shown through the "us vs them" narrative that will be discussed in the next chapter, for instance, by directly attacking or challenging politicians, doctors, or researchers which mediatic visibility: acting as supporters becomes a way to stress their being *against*, depending on the specific case, the medical establishment and the pharmaceutical industry, academic research, or more generally the state and the capitalist society (Lavorgna and Di Ronco, 2017).

In the groups encountered, there are "member hierarchies" depending on frequency of involvement, as well as the perceived quality of that participation (Maratea and Kavanaugh, 2012). In other words, participation to the group tends be "layered," in a combination of both virtual and physical presence opportunities (Licoppe and Inada, 2012) – such as being active supporters online, or attending offline events such as classes and seminars. Many supporters manage to become quite visible and reputable within their networks: by contributing online with remarks of the type admired by the group, their individual reputation is enhanced through a display of identity (Donath, 1996). In turn, their identities (which are built through continuous engagement and, at times, claims of expertise) and their perceived motivations (which need to appear immune from personal gains and ambitions) become very important to create and maintain ingroup trust. Some among the supporters are (less known or visible) providers themselves, or are providers *in fieri* and their participation online becomes a networking (or even "name-dropping") opportunity (*"Thank you to define me [in your post, commenting an essay I wrote among other things] as exceptional… that essay is going to become part of a book, I'll keep you posted"*; *"I learned [non-science-based practice] by attending [name of well-known provider]'s workshops"*). For them, in other words, active participation becomes a way to construct also their professional identity.

3.4. PROVIDERS

By relying on psycho-criminological literature of offender typologies, providers (note: from the specific subgroup of those providing *harmful* non-science-based medical treatments, active in the United Kingdom) were recently categorized into four main types, depending on their prevalent motivations (ranging from the desire to be credited to the presence of strong inner holistic beliefs) or other behavioral determinants (sexual offending or the presence of a mental disorder triggered by a traumatic event) as attainable from documentary sources (Lavorgna and Horsburgh, 2019). The proposed typology includes utilitarian providers, custodial providers (with the subtypes "good-faith" providers and "egotistical fake" providers), sexual abusers, and delusional providers.

First, utilitarian providers are moved mainly by the desire to obtain financial profit; they operate frauds leading to the payment of disproportionate amount of money for useless or even potentially dangerous treatments. Second, custodial providers tend to have a recognized authoritative role and are in a position of power in comparison to their patients, who give them their full trust. Harm, for these providers, is an unwanted by-product of their actions. Particularly "good-faith" providers (often health practitioners, working in modern scientific or alternative health sectors) genuinely believe that they are helping the victim: their moral responsibility lies in overselling the therapeutic value of an alternative treatment, and their criminal responsibility might be framed as a form of negligence. "Egoistical fake" providers, on the contrary, are mainly moved by the desire of receiving validation and legitimation as health authorities, as they have built or are building their whole identity around their work as providers. Third, in a few cases, sexual abusers were identified: a major reason for them to act as providers was to have access to vulnerable victims to sexually abuse them, and the treatment offered was hence a mean to the sexual assault. Fourth, delusional providers are those who believe themselves to be on a mission to heal or to rid their social circles of westernized medicine or "big-pharma" influences, moved by an ideological desire to protect the world from undesirable people.

By looking also at providers' demographic and social characteristics, the same analysis suggested a prevalence of (male) middle-aged adults, and that they become providers in early adulthood. A majority of providers were alternative medicine practitioners (or at least they were presenting themselves as such, see Lavorgna and Horsburgh, 2019 for further details), followed by doctors (most of them running private practices), fake or discredited (former) doctors, "healers," graduates in scientific disciplines, nurses, pharmacists, and yoga teachers. Most providers seemed to be well-integrated in the local communities in which they operated. They tended to operate alone or, when they were part of a group, with autonomy; there was no evidence of structured organizational forms, and networks and associations seemed only as a way to offer one or two providers an aura of legitimacy and sophistication.

The current study has a different scope, and has investigated a diverse range of providers (that is, those engaging in online behaviors, yet not necessarily harmful, targeting an Italian audience and in the midst of the 2020 pandemic). Still, some of its findings seem to confirm those from the British study: when we look at providers, we see a majority of middle-aged males, operating alone, in couples (often with their wives, who at times are providers themselves but with a more limited public visibility) or in small, flexible associations with friends and acquaintances. The declared motivations are, of course, always very positive and constructive (among many others, "*I created this page to help those who want to learn, improve themselves, cure themselves, help, progress, love*"; "*this page offers information, data, ideas and scientific theories*"; "*I think I can make a difference*"; "*this is a project of individual and social evolution*"; "*[this approach] can help those suffering from coronavirus*"; "*[he] decided to write this book to disseminate his enormous knowledge to help and give hope to those suffering*").

However, from the virtual ethnography, the search for financial profit and for validation and legitimation as health authorities were also present. The importance of public validation and, in some cases, the (apparently genuine) attempt to help others (for instance, through spirituality) will be discussed in the next chapter. As regards the search for profit, it is worth noting that in the providers' personal websites it is very common to find links to donate money through PayPal, bank transfers, or even the so-called 5 X 1000 (that is, the share of the taxes to which the Italian State waives in favor of non-profit organizations that you can chose in the tax return). In the personal site of one prominent provider, there is a whole section stressing that he is willing to give talks to symposia and conferences, but for a price, and detailing all his needs that have to be accommodated in order for him to accept an invitation (including: being the only presenter). Both webinars and offline events are costly (from a few dozens to hundreds of Euros). Providers' reputation also becomes a resource for commerce through the advertising of a range of services (including online consultancies on medical issues), health and wellness products (such as vitamins and supplements), books (self-published, or published by a couple of press companies specialized in alternative health practices), or through crowdfunding for various projects (among others, projects to educate children with "high spiritual potential").

As noted in the methodological section, certain providers are very open in presenting online (and, in one case, during the interview) some forms of in-depth autobiographical accounts. From those accounts, a common theme is that they were not satisfied by the "official" medical system, at times as outsiders (that is, they started an alternative path from the outset of their careers) or after having been a part of it for a while (as medicine students, or doctors). Once again, we can generally identify one or more catalyst events that were determinant in their decision to take action and become providers of alternative health practices: these events, similarly to what was observed with supporters, are generally personal crisis (not finding the answers they were looking for) or professional frustration (for instance, an alleged talent or accomplishments not being sufficiently recognized by colleagues, or by the medical establishment).

Providers present or promote a broad range of alternative medical approaches – ranging from those generally recognized by the CAM community (such as homeopathy or Ayurveda) but overselling their effects, to dangerous quackeries with no medical plausibility; others refute scientific findings by proposing alternative interpretations or data (punctually discredited by the scientific community). Education and training for non-conventional practices can be extremely varied. Some of the providers had some forms of conventional training (such as medical or scientific degrees) and then simply developed ideas dismissed by the rest of the scientific community (it might be worth repeating that the cases considered are not about the usual and constructive scientific debates when there is no consolidated scientific agreement, but they pivot around ideas that are not accepted because they completely lack scientific plausibility, or have not been sustained with the standards accepted by the research community of reference). The majority of the providers encountered, however, mention or discuss a range of self-training (from books and online material), informal (ranging from mentoring to "*visiting astral dimensions*"), and formalized training opportunities (weekend courses, but also months-long or years-long programs or "masters" ending with some form of certificate end evaluation), often originating from seeking self-development and improvement, or simply curiosity.

In line with what Alich (2015) lamented when discussing shamanism, this variety of training can be very confusing for the general public, as most people are not aware of this range of educational possibilities and might assume that using a certain title (doctor, homeopath, or even "researcher") implies having gone through a certain uniformity of education and practice. Rather, even in the more formal forms of training flagged by providers, from a quick search on the programs available online it emerges that issues of basic health sciences, as well as ethics, professionalism, and safety are rarely considered (again in line with Alich, 2015).

3.5. CONSPIRATORIAL IDEATION AND EPISTEMIC MISTRUST

In conspiratorial thinking, the existence of a group of agents secretly working together generally for a sinister purpose is postulated; social institutions are ascribed a sort of group personality, and are treated as conspiring agents as if they were individuals (Popper, 1972; Coday, 2006). Conspiratorial thinking and conspiracy-led narratives were observed in the course of the ethnography: some providers and supporters suggest the existence of an alleged system's opposition to alternative health practices, and clandestine governmental plans and other schemes behind major social events, including the pandemic, were discussed (among the more extreme: the allegation that COVID-19 was spread in badly hit parts of Italy through flue jabs; the idea that the new vaccinations will modify our DNA to be then controlled via G5 technology; or the suspicion that a vaccine for COVID-19 is already available but kept secret to the general population for mass control, to impose mandatory vaccines in the near future or to pass repressive or intrusive laws, including the inoculation of microchips). Many – as we will discuss in Section 4.3 – do not trust the government and its use of emergency powers, or the disclosure of personal data; while some of the concerns over the use of emergency powers to allow stronger surveillance mechanisms are legitimate, the conspiratorial element is to be found in the fact that the existence of a clear direction is assumed, and science-fiction elements end up overshadowing realistic alarms on extreme dataveillance (Lettera Aperta, 2020; Lavorgna and Myles, 2021).

Other conspiratorial theories encountered are aligned with QAnon, a cultish right **movement** centering on the central narrative that a "Deep State" cabal of satanic pedophilic global elites are responsible for all the evil in the world. QAnon believers maintained that those same elites were seeking to "bring down" president Trump (see also Section 4.2), seen as the world's only hope to defeat said Deep State (Cosentino, 2020; Amarasingam & Argentino, 2020; McManus et al., 2020; Lavorgna et al., 2021): for instance, when former president Trump tweeted a pro-vaccination statement, a user asked others in the group for *"explanations"*; it was explained to him that was probably a coded message to bring down the Deep State, *"the real virus."*

Conspiratorial thinking and pseudoscience, historically, have always been very close, and they both need to be understood in the context which first allowed to draw some clear lines between the orthodox and the heterodox in epistemological foundations, and the affirmation of "orthodox" intellectuals as the gatekeepers of knowledge in Western countries (see Thalmann, 2019). The term "pseudoscience" started to be used as a sort of offensive and defensive mechanism among scholars in the Cold War culture of the 1950s, and by the end of the following decade conspiracy theories became fully stigmatized in public discourse. Despite this stigmatization in public and scientific discourses, conspiratorial thinking never ceased to speak to people's common sense, and to appeal as a conceptual model. From the 1960s and 1970s, it started to become attractive to those interested in counterculture and counterdiscourses – in a way, the fringe status of conspiracy theories started to become something to capitalize on, something that helps explaining their success still today ("*I am proud of being labelled as a conspiratorial thinker, if that means defending Liberty and Truth*"). Furthermore, even if formally delegitimized, conspiracy theories received continuous media and popular culture attention (treating them as an entertaining selling point), which has familiarized audiences with the contents, making some of these theories quite visible (Thalmann, 2019).

To understand why the pandemic provided such a fertile soil to conspiracy beliefs, it is important to look at individual and group attitudes and behaviors (Biddlestone et al., 2020). Conspiratorial thinking thrives in situations when people's need to feel safe and secure in their world and to exert control over their existence are threatened, as it helps individuals' feelings of agency and power (Imhoff and Lamberty, 2020). Conspiracy theories are often adopted defensively as they offer people some compensatory sense of control, giving them the chance to feel they have some power by rejecting official narratives (Douglas et al., 2020), especially when they need to overcome feelings of alienation or anxiety in times of large-scale social change (Bangerter et al., 2020). Conspiracy theories are also used to relieve individuals from a sense of responsibility for their disadvantaged position. In a way, embracing conspiratorial thinking and looking for purposive explanations where none exists becomes a way to reject the meaningless and Camus-style absurdity-play nature of the social world, the idea that some things "just happen" also when it comes to many politically, culturally, or socially momentous events (Keeley, 1999; Basham, 2001) – as in the case of the pandemic *krisis*, as we will further discuss in the following chapter.

Lack of recognition can be an important factor enabling conspiratorial thinking: indeed, when group members experience relative deprivation or competitive victimhood and end up believing that their ingroup is not given the same opportunities as the outgroup, or that their ingroup has endured more suffering and injustice than the outgroup, conspiracy belief can find a solid basis to grow (Biddlestone et al., 2020). The use of an "us vs them" polarized logic (as will be discussed more in detail in Section 4.2) is key for ingroup identity construction: the antithetic enemy is constructed as a symmetrical copy with a minus sign or a sort of mirror projection of their own model of culture (Leone et al., 2020). Outgroups are stereotyped into two main types: a paternalistic stereotype and feelings of pity are associated with perceptions of the outgroup as warm but incompetent and an envious stereotype and feelings of envy are associated with perceptions of the outgroup as cold but competent (which can generate intergroup resentment toward high-status competitive outgroups) (Biddlestone et al., 2020). Groups associated with the latter stereotypes are those viewed as potential villains – institutionalized science, in the cases observed.

Social psychologists have shown that even if conspiracy theories are often presented by their supporters as rational in nature, they are rather a reflection of certain beliefs about the world, which are in turn the result of a multi-biased information-seeking process (Klein and Nera, 2020). The epistemic authority of modern science is challenged because of three main types of critiques: its alleged dogmatism, the presence of vested interests in scientific knowledge production, and the exclusion of lay knowledge by scientific experts forming a global "elite" (Harabman and Aupers, 2014). As a reaction to this epistemic mistrust, science-related populism – that is, as conceptualized by Mede and Schafer (2020), a set of ideas suggesting the existence of a morally charged antagonism between an (allegedly) virtuous ordinary people and an (allegedly) unvirtuous academic elite – has overtime proposed alternative epistemologies, which can be summed up in attempts to replace established knowledge with different (but still scientific) counterknowledge, and in rejecting the scientific epistemology *tout court* to replace it with common sense, personal experiences, and gut feelings, and promoting an enhanced role of emotions in decision making (see Mede and Schafer, 2020).

In this alternative and experiential knowledge-building process, initial opinions, beliefs, or even self-diagnosis are confirmed and strengthened by communal peer reinforcement. In a sort of social epistemology endeavor, the individuals active in the groups observed seek to pursue the truth with the help of, or in the face of, others. In social epistemology, an individual might look for epistemic help from another agent, or might look for answers by using group members in a collaborative way (Goldman and O'Connor, 2019). Social epistemology, of course, is not negative in itself, and it can be rather used to protect from polluted information (see Goldman and O'Connor, 2019). However, to function properly it needs to be based on sound individual epistemologies – something that often seems to lack at the ingroup level. As a consequence, groups claim that their voices are unheard as they were somehow victims of epistemic injustice (for instance, by claiming that they are not given a voice in public debates because of prejudices about the social group to which they belong) and can be easily dismissed.

Social ties and online communities, through peer reinforcement, have a strong impact on health practices and individualist epistemologies by boosting individuals' confidence in their experiential knowledge: even when group members are not openly endorsing a conspiracy or otherwise non-science-based theory, they might be "liking" them or commenting on them with positive curiosity (in a way, normalizing them), and preferring them to the scientifically supported explanations, when available (Mirable and Horne, 2019; Lavorgna and Myles, 2021). In this context, information is denied or dismissed on the basis of mechanisms such as confirmation bias (people tend to perceive and interpret new information in a way that confirms their original beliefs while ignoring or rejecting information that contradicts those beliefs), myside bias (people tend to evaluate and generate evidence that helps to confirm their own opinions), and belief perseverance (people will cling to their original beliefs, even when confronted with credible evidence to the contrary) (Stanovich et al., 2013; Peruzzi et al., 2019; Prot and Anderson 2019). For instance, traditional media are harshly attacked (as "*sell-outs*") when they report stories of young people dying or getting severely sick from the virus (as this not aligned with their idea that "*only old people get sick*"). Furthermore, these patterns are facilitated by specific narrative mechanisms used to strengthen intragroup community and undermine scientific evidence (Duchsherer et al., 2020).

Conspiratorial ideation tends to rely on two main communicative genres: storytelling (narratives tend to display plot elements similar to dramatized stories featuring the actions of heroes, villains and the like and their goals) and argumentation (when supporters and skeptics debate a particular version of the events) (Bangerter et al., 2020). Storytelling is successful as it allows to craft a sense of community, creating a common space (Duchsherer et al., 2020). Argumentation, through a number of strategies – such as source-related fallacies (*ad populum, ad verecundiam,* and *ad hominem*), analogies, hasty generalizations, and shifts in the burden of proof – allows to attack the unaccepted official version, without entering into the details of the conspiracy theory supported (Oswald, 2016; Bangerter et al., 2020). Interestingly, Hristov (2019) relies on the rhetoric concept of parrhesia (Foucault, 2001) – that is, a figure of speech consisting in speaking candidly or asking forgiveness for so speaking – to problematize the nexus of knowledge, power, and truth affecting conspiratorial thinking, situating this issue in a broader context of unequal social structures. According to Hristov, conspiracy theorists are discursive revolutionaries (even if weak ones, as they do not articulate an alternative social order) who make impossible knowledge claims because they suffer, and their suffering has social roots: they want to cover a lack of meaning in the social order. They turn to parrhesiastic claims which belong to the realm of spirituality rather than to the one of facts (positive knowledge), being grounded in a regime of truth that can be reached only by "true subjects," committed to transform themselves through reflection, experience, and committed work on oneself. In other words, conspiracy theories do not provide statements about facts but rather acts of speech determined by the desire to tell the truth against the powerful, but that fall short of reaching that aim (Hristov, 2019, p. 93).

We have already mentioned how supporters and providers do not rely on official (and often better regulated) channels of publication, but are rather distributed through personal websites and social media, which tend to be considerably less regulated (Thalmann, 2019). Furthermore, cyberspace does not only facilitate the replication and diffusion of certain content, but rather fosters its reinterpretation and personalization through the possibility to sample, remix, or remake content is a way that provokes both users' engagement and agency (Stano, 2020). Even if to different extents, receivers and supporters do not "just read" information on traditional or social media; they tend to be a productive audience actively exploiting diverse types of media as a cultural resource to build a coherent narrative of their worldview and construct their identity, tapping into various fragments of texts, audiovisual material, scientific facts, and literary fiction. As stressed by Aupers (2020), in conspiratorial thinking videos produced and shared on platforms such as YouTube are of particular interest as these videos are often an assemblage of a selection and careful combination of textual, visual, and audio fragments and cues presented (often with a voice-over explanation of what is "really" going on provided by the author) to build a coherent and convincing narrative. The visual elements are key, as they allow for a sort of "virtual eye-witnessing," in line with the motto that "seeing is believing," that allows and reinforces the oppositional reading of mass media events (Aupers, 2020). For instance, of particular interest in this regard was the video showing European politicians allegedly wearing masks only for official photos; their voices were not heard, but (fake) subtitles were added to suggest that these politicians were making joke of those wearing masks. Also, the posting of interviews to providers and known (within the community) supporters from private television channels or through real time or prerecorded videos is quite common.

4

BUILDING IDENTITIES AND NETWORKS THROUGH CONVERGING FRAMES

4.1. INTRODUCTION

Despite the heterogeneity of the participants observed, there are some major underlying themes and narrative frames that can be identified (Kaptchuk and Eisenberg, 1998). As we will see, these themes and frames independently push diverse (but converging and compatible) discourses, facilitating socialization with what are perceived as like-minded people by structuring intragroup attitudes and beliefs, but also facilitating their engagement with a larger audience.

As already noted in the previous chapter, the online presentation of providers (but also of many supporters) is carefully constructed, showing how they desire to appear (Donath, 1996), which in itself can be very revealing (Goffman, 1959). The first part of this chapter presents some of the main narrative frames that inform the "narratives of the self" (Gergen and Gergen, 1983) as emerging through this study. We will see that identities are built through interplay of tensions and dichotomies, crafting social imaginaries and imaginaries of the self that can be very diverse if taken singularly, but that are nonetheless connected by some major converging themes. As such, even if we cannot distinguish a specific or clearly defined subculture, in line with social identity theory, we can notice how behavior is linked to the group's social identity, being more than a collection of individuals behaving *en masse*; individuals are influenced by group identity, for instance, by being motivated to protect and enhance the positivity of their group to establish positive ingroup status or ingroup distinctiveness in order to protect and enhance their own self-esteem (Hogg, 2016; Martiny and Rubin, 2016).

The frames informing these "narratives of the self" pivot around the image of themselves (such as "experts," "belonging," and "free/libertarian") that the participants observed want to project to others and which are at the basis of their online socialization. There are other narrative frames, however, that are commonly found but that respond to in a subtler way to participants' use of the social media groups to find not only support and reassurance among like-minded people, but also a sense of agency, of control over their lives. Online interactions, in a way, become an important tool allowing the agential self to further practices of freedom, ethics of self-care, and a self-oriented morality (Foucault, 1988). This latter aspect, which will be explored in the second part of this chapter, cannot be overlooked if we want to understand why certain misinformation is popular and successful: the narratives offered in our networks of interest are not only persuasive, but they are restorative to some, enabling some participants to find a renewed sense of the self and purpose (Kaptchuk and Eisenberg, 1998; Lavorgna and Myles, 2021).

4.2. NARRATIVES OF THE SELF

4.2.1. I am the Expert!

Providers self-define themselves as experts (for instance, as doctors, scientists, coaches, and even *"world leader"* of a specific pseudoscientific field), and supporters and receivers follow them because of their (perceived) expert or quasi-expert role. This is not surprising, as much of the social dimension of non-science-based practices depends on the fact that they are based on the power, or charisma, of providers (Barcan, 2015). At the same time, some of the supporters attempt to become themselves recognized as expert in the context of their social networks, probably in the attempt to get more recognition and status in the online group (Lavorgna and Myles, 2021). Researchers have already shown how cyberspace and its convergent technologies, in combination with a neoliberal environment somehow incentivizing exaggeration and over-glamorization in self-promotion, have given individuals without recognized qualifications a platform for potentially large-scale communication, where they can construct a cleansed version of themselves, using digital storytelling and curated narratives to take a role that was once reserved for highly trained specialists (Khamis et al., 2016; Rojek, 2017; Lavorgna and Sugiura, 2019).

Unfortunately, the identity clues and proxy indicators that a trained researcher can be used to identify a fake expert more or less easily (for instance, publications and appearances in predatory journals and conferences, flawed methodologies, lack of disciplinary expertise, lack of training in research method, and rational thinking) might be difficult to check for the general public. In their expert role, providers insinuate doubts on the "official" information, and offer their alternative interpretations, thesis, or hypotheses ("*We need to verify whether this news is true, however…*"). Often these are merely conjectures that are nonetheless presented as proofs or demonstrations: the line of reasoning followed sounds reasonable and deserving of trust (Lavorgna and Myles, 2021). Hence, a fake expert might be posing as an expert for a long time before being called out as a fraud (Donath, 1996). Furthermore, even when they are identified as non-expert or frauds by the scientific or medical communities, this fact in most cases does not affect their online presence and standing, their narrative, or supporters' activities and behaviors. Providers, indeed, simply lament the fact that they are denied a place in the debate, conversely of what they identify as their nemesis, coming from the "official" science ("*we were prevented from analyzing the bodies of those dead because of the new coronavirus*"). They present themselves as martyrs, or paladins of "*true research.*" This attitude characterizes the so-called science-related populism, where the scientific elites are portrayed as antagonists of the ordinary people: they are seen as morally inferior, and considered collectively as the power-force making all science-related decisions such as agendas, methods, and publications to produce what is supposed to be "true" knowledge but that is in fact elusive, contested, and detached from the everyday life of ordinary people (Mede and Schafer, 2020). As such, science-related populism challenges organized science, and questions the way in which science produces knowledge and therefore, ultimately, its authority to support science-based decision making (in what is perceived, in a derogative way, as a "*scientocracy*") (see also Collins and Evans, 2008).

Interestingly, in crafting "expert" identities, even if "science" (or, to be more precise, institutionalized science) is not trusted by many in the groups observed, the use of scientific and academic imaginaries is common among most supporters to be seen as reputable, giving credibility to their claims. Providers and supporters are prodigious in providing information online, generally posting links to poor sources of information as if they are credible: beyond referring to bogus or predatory scientific journals (that might appear legitimate to the general public) or predatory (as it emerges from quick online checks) conferences as mentioned above, they refer – among other things – to collaborations with (unrecognized) universities, or "studies" that do not present empirical data, or lack sufficient methodological details. If they spent some time (for instance, as students) in a well-known or prestigious university, that relationship is amplified, for instance, suggesting to their audience that they have or had an affiliation there. When data are discussed, they are often presented visually to prove a point, but generally in a partial and misleading way. The fact that this type of "evidence" is generally accepted by supporters and receivers is an important factor in perpetuating the cycle of science denial and the sharing of potentially dangerous misinformation. Science-sounding names are used (with *"quantum"* and *"energy"* being unsurprisingly very common, see Gazzola, 2019). Providers and supporters belonging to the same social networks have put together a "parallel system" of alternative workshops, seminars, and similar events that are often referred to as a way to show scientific status (*"frontier scientific research"*).

The attempt to look sciency is reinforced through visual elements. In posted pictures, videos, and webinars, providers (generally middle-aged or senior white men, in rarer cases middle-aged white women) present themselves in serious yet approachable settings (for instance, indoor in a living room, a small studio with books, or in front of a white board or a microscope, or at times outdoor in a calm, green space; white lab coats are often used – see also Lavorgna and Myles, 2021); their body language, appearance, and tone are relaxed.

Some historical science figures, and Galileo above all, have a myth-like status: they fought the good fights, and promoters like to compare themselves to them. Galileo, with his book, did a deliberate act of transgression, unleashing the wrath of the Inquisition; the subversive implications of his act made him a sort of hero of modern science. Aligning themselves to Galileo's iconic story, providers and supporters have a pride in describing themselves as *"transgressive,"* *"heretics,"* *"dissidents,"* *"free thinkers,"* or *"against the current."* By doing this, a false dichotomy of science is furthered, opposing providers – that is, those allegedly following a truly open, free, and inquisitive research – to the *"sellouts,"* *"arrogant"* scientists with an hidden agenda, belonging to the *"scientific papacy."*

4.2.2. Outgroup Hostility and Ingroup Belonging

As anticipated above, providers complain that their voices are not heard, that they are silenced or censored by the system, which is bent over the interest of – depending on the group – the pharmaceutical sector, the European Union and foreign governments, or the hidden (Satanist) elites ruling the world. By opposing themselves – and, consequently, their supporters and followers – to these negative forces, promoters actively contribute to build and strengthen a sense of group identity, promoting a strong "us vs them," oppositional narrative (*"this is a fight of good vs evil,"* *"we are the sons of Light, they are the sons of Darkness"*). Being an outsider (like the transgressive Galileo) becomes an element of pride: as self-perception of personal behavior is influenced by the emotional and cultural capital coming from social interactions, through the online community a (potentially) stigmatized identity can then be turned into a positive one (Maratea and Kavanaugh, 2012). Using the fringe status as a marketing tool, certain promoters offer "identifying connections" for those who comparably perceive themselves as alienated or rejected by mainstream culture (Thalmann, 2019, p. 13).

On the contrary, the sharp distinction vs "them" is maintained and reinforced constantly. In line with social identity processes (McCoy and Major, 2003; Brewer, 2007) and intergroup threat theory (Stephan et al., 2002; Prot and Anderson, 2019), members of the community react in a defensive and often hostile manner when the perspective of outsiders is reported, as a way to protect the ingroup worldview. Similarly, when encountering health information and communication that depicts them negatively, threatening their self-image and perceive worth, because of defensiveness (Prot and Anderson, 2019) individuals react by lowering their perceptions of risk as a mechanism for self-affirmation. The use of insulting or derogatory terms, as well as the use of ridicule and humor (see Fig. 4.1), are important elements in the

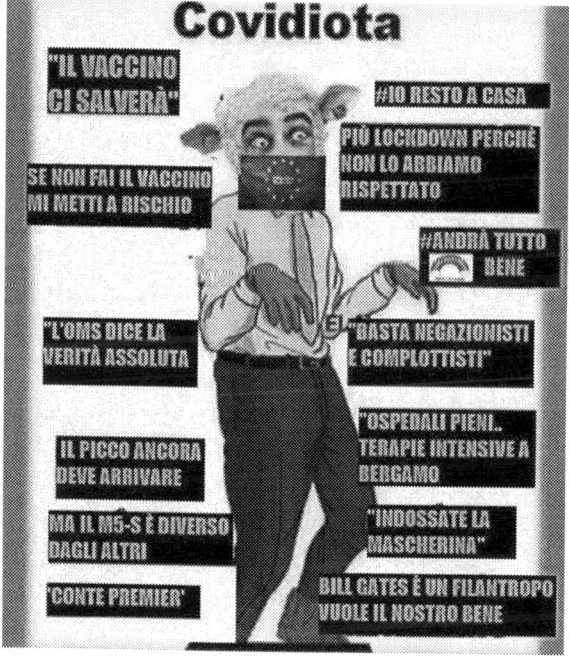

Fig. 4.1. Meme on Inverted "Covidiots".
[Translation: "The vaccine will save us"; "if you do not vaccine yourself, you will put me at risk"; "the WHO always says the truth"; "the peak has not arrived yet"; "The 5-Stars Movement is different"; "premier Conte"; "#istayhome"; "more lockdown as we did not complied with it"; "everything will be fine"; "no more negationists and conspiratorial thinkers," "hospitals are full ... intensive care in Bergamo"; "put your masks on"; "Bill Gates is a philanthropist and operates for our good"].

construction of a counternarrative, here used as a form of critique targeting members of what are perceived by these users as members of a social outgroup. For instance, while "covidiot" has been used as an insulting term for those ignoring health advice about COVID-19, within the ingroup the meaning is reversed: "covidiots" are those following the governmental preventive measures, and "believing" – among other things – in the WHO (OMS in Italian), vaccines, and the philanthropic work of Mr Gates as exemplified in the meme below.

According to the largely predominant ingroup view, risks are somehow exaggerated or constructed by those with power to manipulate people (*"they try to gaslight people into the* [anti-COVID-19] *vaccine"*; "*coronavirus is a global coup d'état*"), and those falling for this are labeled as "*a flock of sheep enslaved to the regime*," "*parrots*," "*lobotomized*," "*gullible*," "*addicted [to their fake reality]*," "*indoctrinated*," or "*psychotic*."

If the imaginary associated to science and research is positive when linked to the providers, conversely, the esthetic associated to what they consider to be "bad science" (consider, for instance, the anonymized screenshot from a video suggested that COVID-19 was engineered in a Chinese laboratory, here reported as Fig. 4.2) is a stereotypization of science as something cold, mechanical, abstruse: the images used (some of which from the 2011 move *Contagion*) are dark, upsetting (for instance, claustrophobic spaces, with people wearing face covers and masks), or grotesque; in videos, over-the-top dramatic or angsty music is used. Interesting, in the earliest stages of the pandemic, images showing people covered with masks were often showing people with Asian traits, inserted in discourses suggesting this was a "foreign" virus, attacking Italian lifestyle.

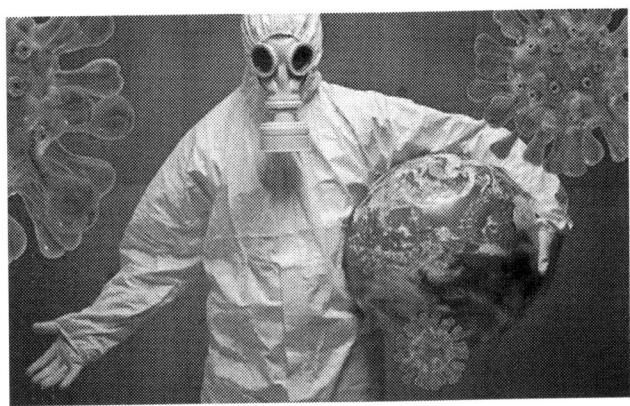

Fig. 4.2. Bad Scientists.

Identity construction and the search for recognition within the group is a key motivator for taking part in online discussions. Participants are supposed to be sympathetic to the core ideas around which the group is based, as they are at the very basis of the social identity of the group (Donath, 1996). Sometimes this can be as simple as repeated affirmations ("*Yes, I agree!*") emphasizing the affiliation to a certain idea, or person – specific promoters and supporters, in our case. Depending on the nature of the group and the other parts to the conversation, individual participation can manifest itself by posting rude flames or cutting observations to "defend" the values and the "truths" presented in the group from outsiders or divisive voices, or rather by providing a polite answer to a query, which is seen as a way to contribute to the group (ingroup altruism is generally expected or encouraged). Indeed, identity building is a pivotal concept also in providing ingroup support: those recognized as genuine community members are never belittled or alienated; rather, an inclusive language ("*we*") is generally used, and reassurance, support, and empathy are looked for ("*I have been alone for a lifetime, no one wanted me*") and offered (for instance, the providers make often reference to the common fears and anxieties, especially financial, suffered by many during the lockdowns – see also Lavorgna and Myles, 2021). The more individuals feel to belong to a certain group (for instance, very active members), the more they express group emotions in strong ways, hence motivating and regulating ingroup behaviors (Mackie et al., 2000; Smith et al., 2007).

If belonging to the group (the "us") has certainly a core role in defining the (at least online) persona of promoters and supporters, milder supporters and other participants are also very keen in asserting their individual selves, while being an integrated part of larger wholes because of their systems of values and beliefs. This balance is manifested also in the esthetic sought: for example, in the wave of the new sets of restrictions taking place in Autumn 2020, with a new surge in hospitalizations across the country and masks made mandatory again in public places, some supporters started to suggest to use a symbol on the mask – a sun – to escape anonymization and to reassert a certain "*way of thinking,*" while allowing to recognize like-minded people in a way that they could then "*make their smiles meet*" (suggesting that they could then both agree to take their masks off).

For most individuals taking part in the groups observed there is no clear indication of social, political, or even ideological homogeneity, even if some converging narratives – as we will soon discuss – can be identified. Furthermore, the frequency, duration, and intensity of participation in online discussion varies tremendously. Consequently, rather than being isolated from the discussions occurring elsewhere, many participants present into their (transient, situational) ingroup a broad range of personal social networks (for instance, references to significant others) and experiences (such as discussions occurred in other physical or online social networks, or viewpoints of individuals not belonging to the group, see Lavorgna and Myles, 2021).

Goldsmith and Brewer (2015) stressed in their work on digital drift that when we look at more qualitative data in detail we often notice that many studies looking at organizational structures tend to overlook the role of individual choices, and social and situational contexts. Indeed, contrary to what is suggested by recent big data analyses pointing toward the presence of well-formed and segregated communities (see, for instance, Del Vicario et al., 2016), when we look closer at the online debates and the individuals populating them we see that this representation holds true only for a vocal minority at the core of these networks. Rather, manual, qualitative analysis indicates that participants in the online communities observed are extremely heterogeneous, and bring in and out of the alternative and counterinformation communities of interest all type of information, spreading health-related pollution while not being able to counter it because of the ingroup peer-led mechanisms for sufficiently aligned content to maintain the social identity of the group.

As such, common metaphors such as "echo chambers" and "filter bubbles," when applied to health-related polluted information, might convey the misleading idea that we are dealing with closed systems, and that the problem of mis/dis-information might somehow be "fixed" via algorithmic manipulation addressing named online hotspots that are enabling users to be surrounded by like-minded people and information congruent with their existing beliefs (Artime et al., 2020). However, when we zoom in and look closely at the social reality, it appears that any solution cannot overlook confronting the crisis of trust in contemporary society, and the necessity to incentivize a widespread culture change (Mason et al., 2020). Technical or human intervention on specific social media that do not take into sufficient account the in/out group relations only risk to make certain discussions subterranean phenomena, displacing them into more private social media and therefore making them less accessible for research and targeted interventions. In certain discussion threads there were links to chats on WhatsApp and Telegram, and an interviewee confirmed that their group was increasingly preferring these means of communications to avoid intrusions from outsiders.

4.2.3. Politics of (Negative) Liberties

While most participants observed do not side themselves politically, some are very vocal supporters of political parties or movements, and some are political actors themselves. In Italy, notable is the case of the 3V Movement, a political party *"for the freedom of choice"* dedicated to the abolition of mandatory vaccination (it presents itself on social media as *"the only political movement asking for the Truth and putting human wellness and health at the core of their political action"*) who entered the political arena in 2019 and that in late 2020 organized public demonstrations against the *"medical dictatorship"* and the preventive and harm-mitigation measures adopted during the pandemic. Elsewhere in the ethnography, other self-defined movements *"of resistance"* or *"civil disobedience"* were identified, such as one named after the modern Latin phrase *vi veri veniversum vivus vici* ("by the power of truth, I, while living, have conquered the Universe"), popularized by the graphic novel and the movie "V for Vendetta": according to some of its members, *"we are in a war, but we are not fighting against a virus, but against the attempt to take our liberties away from us."*

Regardless of the explicit embracement of a certain political party or movement, however, political sensitive themes at times (in fora focusing on health) or very often (in fora self-defined as "counterinformation") emerge, providing important insights on the system of values and ideologies of the participants observed. Overall, the pandemic has supplied fertile ground for sovereigntist, antigovernment, and radical right movements (Lavorgna et al., 2021), who have somehow joined forces with conspiracy theorists in online debates and anticontainment protests across the country, in a way that resembles the alignment between the antivax movement and Italy's populist parties (Massa, 2019). Similarly to what has been observed in the United States (Lavorgna et al., 2021), the themes raised are very diverse, ranging from election politics (for instance, attacking the prime minister Conte and other Italian politicians as *"traitors,"* while praising – though only in some groups – president Trump and commenting the American elections as fraudulent) to social control (for instance, comparing the face masks to those worn by slaves, or to muzzles), from issues of (lost) sovereignty and anti-European narratives (*"The are selling us to Germany and China"*) to issues of ethnicity and immigration (for instance, commenting on refugees arriving via boat in late Summer in Southern Italy: *"at the beginning of the pandemic we had sick people, and were importing masks; now we have masks, and are importing sick people"* – see also Fig. 4.3). In an identity-building perspective, the prevailing sentiment of suspicion and mistrust toward both immigrants and other countries is not surprising when we read this in the context of the discontent arising out of the material and ontological uncertainties and relative deprivation engendered by globalization (Young, 2003): blaming and negatively essentializing others, from this perspective, is an integral part of the process of reaffirming and hardening one's cultural identity.

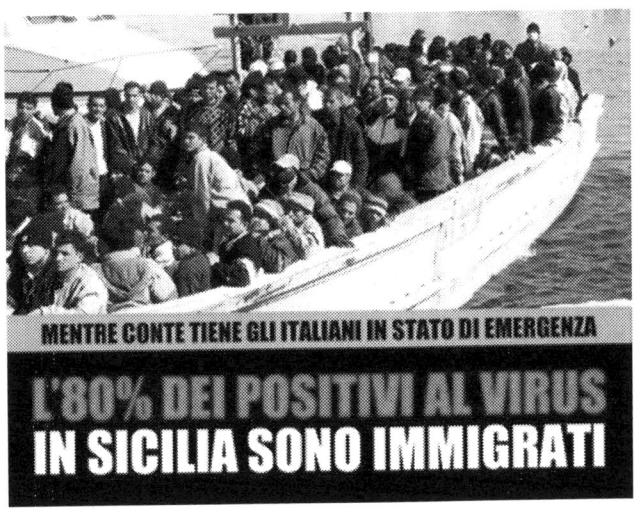

Fig. 4.3. They are Infecting Us.
[Translation: While Conte (the Italian Prime Minister in 2020, a.n.) keeps the Italians in a state of emergency, 80% of those positive to the virus in Sicily are immigrants].

Again in a logic of "us vs them," the transversal theme of *freedom* (vs the government, the European Union or, in general, power elites) is what brings together the narratives encountered, allowing very diverse actors – some acting in their individual capacity, others as part of a specific movement or organization – to independently promote diverse (but politically compatible, and converging under the same transversal theme) discourses. This freedom, however, is a very specific one: it is the one related to the *negative liberties* (that is, the absence of constraints) of individual agents (rather than the collectives' possibility of acting to realize one's fundamental purposes), in line with contemporary right-wing and populist libertarian views (Boaz, 2008) and ideas of self-reliance (and often minimal government). These ideologies and cultural worldview play an important role in science denial and in the opposition to preventive measures such as lockdowns, limitations to traveling and gathering, and the use of masks, which are here seen as an undue interference impacting individual and group liberties. In line with the psychological mechanisms of reactance (Prot and Anderson 2019), scientific evidence is rejected when perceived as a threat to personal freedom.

In Italy, the populist rhetoric (also in its libertarian form), in its encounter and partial convergence with a nationalist ideology, has frequently embraced a controversial form of moral and religious conservatism on civil liberties' matters like abortion and same-sex marriages, while opposing the attitude of (part of) the Church, including Pope Francis, toward immigrants – in line with some Protestant religious groups in the United States (Martinelli, 2018). In line with these views, it is not surprising that in the (overall rare) posts and discussion where – for instance – gender issues are discussed, a libertarian form of feminist (Sommers, 1994) or attacks toward what is dismissed as "*gender feminism*" are prevalent; women are recognized as political peers but a traditional vision of the family, with a gendered division of roles, is advocated ("*First of all, a mother*"). The LGBTQ community is disdained ("*Natural family [...] is in the order of things*"), even if on this latter point views are more openly divided.

4.3. AGENCY AND EMPOWERMENT

4.3.1. My Body, My Self

By being part of a group, individuals who experienced a (at least perceived) loss of agency and choice can re-establish a sense of control (Matza, 1964, 1969). Through this affiliation to a certain group, the subject engages in a continuous creation and adaptation of the meaning of a certain behavior, and of self-identity (Haines, 1981). In this perspective, the empowering aspects of cyberspace have already been stressed in the literature (Goldsmith and Brewer, 2015), but it is important to stress that the constant reassertion of agency and the related rejection of any perceived form of authority and judgment goes beyond online avatars and appears deeply rooted in a system of beliefs that extends, for instance, to pedagogical philosophies: for example, some providers and supporters posted links to recommended camps for children and their families; home education and Steinerian schools are approved, while nurseries for small children are not.

In the context of the pandemic, many experienced a loss of agency in the crisis; by siding with groups promoting the idea that control can be taken back ("*join us if you are a warrior!*"; "*we repudiate this system based on fear!*"), they are trying to regain a sense of power (an attitude that political and extremist movements embracing the #NoMask umbrella have learnt to exploit very well, as discussed in Lavorgna et al., 2021). This idea of re-establishing control finds a proper soil in the alternative health environment, where an emphasis on individual responsibility in terms of health is prevalent – from trying to prevent diseases through a healthy lifestyle, to considering themselves somehow responsible when they get sick (Martin and Debons, 2015). Indeed, some of the advice provided in the groups observed genuinely promotes a healthy lifestyle, as individuals are encouraged to take agency upon their lives by eating healthily, exercising, and living *"positively."* The harms come when some of the information provided is potentially very dangerous, and promoting risky behaviors.

In terms of pandemic-specific advices, it is often implied that the use of masks is unnecessary (some users mention not to use them, or to take layers off; others are among the active promoters of antimasks gatherings; in the early stages of the pandemic, videos were posted with groups of friends and families, including children, setting masks to fire); that hand washing is useless if not potentially negative for the health if carried out as advised by official health advisors; that physical distancing is useless, as the virus is *"a fake pandemic," "not existing," "dead," "just a light flue"* (and, indeed, some users were referring to participation to events were distancing was not respected, even posting pictures); and that "cures" are already available but kept hidden (in a few instances very perilous suggestions were given, such as to use bleach). Some groups offer a range of antimask self-certification modules or lockdown movement permits ready for download (updated as the governmental guidelines changed), and also *"legal advice"* as well as *"medical advice"* (non-better specified). Those "at-risk" (that is, those more vulnerable because of age of pre-existing conditions) are othered (Douglas, 1992), and somehow marginalized to mainstream society in the narrative of risk (Brown, 2020). The number of deaths is minimized, trivialized. In other words, preventive and responsive measures are opposed as they are seen as an instrument of social and institutional control, as *"much ado about nothing."* Interestingly, however, enlisting individuals in the pursuit of self-improvement and autonomy could also be interpreted as a way to control and govern them, consistently with neo-liberalist ideas of a hyper-responsible self, with the individual held responsible for success or failure, health or sickness (Rimke, 2000).

Consistently with the idea of maintaining agency and control over their lives and bodies, and with the lack of trust toward medical information coming from the government or from outgroup experts, it is not surprising that the communities observed are aligned with antivax beliefs (some, indeed, were openly antivax, publishing, for example, photos and stories of children allegedly "killed" by vaccines): they refuse to *"become the guinea pigs of an experimental vaccine,"* and denounce the potential creation of a prospective *"cast system, based on vaccinations."* Those with more extreme views do not hesitate to call COVID-19 vaccines *"crimes against the humanity,"* comparing them to *"experiments in Auschwitz"* carried out by a *"Nazi state."* When the primrose started to be used as a symbol for the vaccinations in Italy (with the slogan "Italy is reborn with a flower"), a small community started to compare the flower with Jewish badges.

4.3.2. Spirituality

For some of the groups observed, spirituality is the key theme around which individuals pivot. Spirituality or spiritual belief, it is worth recalling, has to do with an individual's search for existential meaning and is not necessarily linked to religion (which is one way to express spiritual belief through a framework of rituals, codes, and practices) (Tanyi, 2002; Speck et al., 2004). Spirituality has been recognized as an important, positive factor contributing to wellbeing and coping strategies (Koenig et al., 1999; Speck et al., 2004), and as such it is not surprising to see it linked to health-related discourses, or used as a mechanism for personal empowerment. In several social media pages (and – interestingly – in many individual comments posted in groups that do not have a spiritualistic focus), it was relatively common to find inspirational posts, images (especially with references to angelology) and videos, or spiritualist prayers, providing support and reassurance toward death and illness, but most of all toward the social and economic uncertainties of the pandemic. In this context, spirituality is often presented as a mechanism for personal empowerment (or "*awakening*"): there are multiple messages coming from both the providers (through posts and videos) and those commenting that, while discussing spiritual matters, encourage people to take agency and control over their own body and mind – for instance, by strengthening the spirit by viewing the pandemic as a time for personal growth (see also Lavorgna and Myles, 2021).

Problematically, however, in many cases spiritualism was presented as in opposition to science-based approaches ("*Science is the devil*") that are viewed as incompatible with the intuition-based form of knowledge that much spiritualism promotes. This is in line with research (carried out in the more secularized cultural context of the Netherlands) suggesting that contemporary spirituality is a key contributor to science skepticism, to the point that is a better predictor than religiosity when it comes, for instance, to skepticism about vaccination, low faith in science, and unwillingness to support science (Rutjens and van der Lee, 2020).

4.3.3. Privacy and Self-disclosure

The value of privacy, and more in general the importance to protect personal data, seem to be a matter of concerns of most participants, which frame this issue as a corollary of retaining their freedoms and maintain control on their selves. In the virtual ethnography, it was very common to find participants expressing fears to be "*spied,*" and that "*something*" was hidden to them when discussing, for instance, the use of the contact tracing app Immuni (that is, the official exposure notification app of the Italian government), the need to provide credentials and contact details upon mandatory testing when returning to Italy from abroad, and the need of emergency power by the government. Similarly, during the attempts to carry out the narrative interviews, many refused to sign the mandatory consent forms mentioning "privacy concerns" (see Lavorgna and Sugiura, 2020). Some participants try to take control over what they perceive as unwelcomed incursions and attacks hindering their right to privacy, and present themselves as active in "*committees*" to defend truth and freedom.

This strenuous defense of privacy, however, is in tension with the publication in the open web of personal information. On the platforms encountered, for instance, apart from a minority of participants that were clearly using aliases and fantasy names (in contrast with the real-name policy of social media companies such as Facebook), the majority of participants were identifiable online with their full names, and many of their personal pages were open to the public. Furthermore, also very private information, including the discussion of sensitive health information regarding participants' themselves or family members, were openly discussed.

Researchers have already stressed how, with the development of the ubiquitous cyberspace and social media in it, also discourses traditionally linked to a private sphere (such as those health-related) have increasingly become a public experience (Conrad et al., 2016), and especially "light" social media users tend to have relaxed privacy attitudes online (Tsay-Vogel et al., 2018). During the ethnography, it was interesting to note how self-disclosure in many cases got the upper hand with privacy concerns, and that dimensions of vertical (institutional) privacy were of much more concern to the individuals observed than dimensions of horizontal privacy (that is, privacy between users of social media platforms) (in opposition to the more general findings of Quinn et al., 2019), suggesting that vertical privacy concerns are a characterizing feature of the communities observed.

5

DRIFTING OFF THE POLLUTED PATHWAY

5.1. CONTEXTS OF CROSSDISCIPLINARITY

This study has furthered a sociological approach to pandemics, in line with previous studies which have recognized pandemics as social problems by looking at how they are perceived, their regulatory institutional structures, or by considering issues on body vulnerability, processes of stigmatization and marginalization, structural inequalities, and health efforts to detect and pre-empt disease spread (French et al., 2018). In this case, however, the focus has been on some socio-cultural processes enabling and sustaining the propagation of potentially harmful (mis)information during the current coronavirus pandemic. The topics of polluted information and medical misinformation are not traditional or mainstream criminological ones, and have been so far relatively overlooked in the social sciences more in general. I have argued, however, that colleagues from the social sciences and specifically criminology should consider them within their "academic jurisdiction," in light of the social harms these behaviors allow – even if this means stretching, and looking beyond, some strict disciplinary boundaries. After all, because of their interstitial character (Abbott, 2001), the social sciences tend to occupy spaces between disciplines and often overlap other disciplinary spaces; criminology in particular has already shown a structural capacity for adaptation, proving able to expand its focus to maintain its relevance (Zedner, 2007).

In the context of online social harms, looking beyond strict disciplinary boundaries can be very useful from the outset in identifying emerging issues – it is not unusual that social harms are revealed through the work of activists, journalists, and scholars in other disciplines (Pemberton, 2007) – as well as in defining appropriate methodological approaches.

Methodologically, this study mostly relied on passive virtual ethnography, which limits the researcher in considering a relatively small sample of potentially relevant material, with implications for data generalizability. Also, to better account for relevant socio-cultural elements, data are conceptualized, interpreted, and integrated in an open iterative process, meant to provide a well-founded and congruent interpretation of the data grounded in the data themselves (Braun et al., 2019), rather than aiming at providing standards of rigor defined in terms of falsifiability and reproducibility. Yet despite these limitations, as discussed in Section 2.2, it is important to stress the necessity to retain space, also in online research, for qualitative analyses that do not aim at ultimate laws, but still can offer relevant meanings through interpretation. In a (media-reinforced) social context too often overlooking or dismissing the social sciences and the humanities, propagating popular ideas about the nature of research as only based on positivistic approaches relying on quantitative, experimental, or statistical methods (Cassidy, 2014), I wanted to make the case for "zooming in" non-probability sampled and relatively small datasets that can nonetheless offer rich and detailed insights to complex social problems; and for approaches that recognize the "contested, blurred, ambiguous, and unsuited for quantification" (Hayward and Young, 2004, p. 114) nature of certain research, opposing the false sense of mathematical precision through quantification that is created in computational investigations of polluted information and medical misinformation online, in a dangerous push toward reductionism. In this study we have unpacked the role of online socialization and identity construction in explaining the nature and success of medical misinformation. But without digging below the surface of network interactions, it could have been more difficult to connect the propagation of harmful misinformation (also during the current pandemic crisis), for instance, to the deep identity crisis suffered by some that can be traced back to some globalization's spillovers; or to the relative deprivation experienced in the "bulimic society" (as described by Young, 2003, p. 394) preaching the liberal mantra of freedom but practicing exclusion, and creating to some a constant feeling of being disrespected, overlooked, and humiliated. We have observed how individuals drift in and out exposure to polluted information in their online experience, but also noticed how they drift online and offline. As stressed by Webber and Yip (2013), this second type of drift is very important to help us to overcome the determinism proper of more positivistic accounts, which focuses on the online presence, and the online relationships, of our individuals of interest, simplifying their "messy humanity" (p. 199) up to the point that we risk losing the diversity and dynamism of the social reality under investigation.

Having said this, in the perspective of future research, pragmatist research approaches using mixed methods are to be welcomed, as they offer a way to allow to address the shortcomings of both positivistic and constructivist research, while taking the best from both worlds (Maruna, 2010; Tinati et al., 2012; Halford et al., 2018; Berendt et al., 2020). Indeed, online social harms – and, among those, information pollution and medical misinformation – are topics that favor interdisciplinary approaches to make good use of both technical abilities to look at large datasets to allow for results' generalizability, and of the capacity to contextualize data into broader complex societal arenas. In other words, both computational and qualitative expertise are essential to progress with cyberspace research and understanding, while maintaining our individual rights and the public good in the digital age (Lavorgna, 2021b). In working with cyberspace (as a data source or analytical resource), social scientists have a toolbox of non-positivistic methods which are precious resources to build knowledge (Halford et al., 2013). In genuine interdisciplinary research, these methods retain a proper space, as positivistic and constructivist standpoints can work together utilizing a broad range of complementary methodologies to garner deeper insights, depending on the specific research questions.

Of course, integrating approaches that draw on intellectual and methodological insights from different disciplines is not something easy to be implemented, as this requires a serious effort in understanding other disciplines' language, theoretical and methodological frameworks, and standards – which may vary considerably, as epistemologies at the very basis of different disciplines are at times, at least apparently, not well aligned, making it difficult to fully integrate them. The effort, however, is worth it. Reflecting on the use of social media data, which can offer important new avenues for research but also needs to be dealt with critically (especially as regards potential biases and the unknown provenance of some data), Halford et al. (2018) argued for the need of a socio-technical approach: data do not exist in the wild and are not discovered, but they are rather *constructed* as objects/subjects of knowledge; as such, "harvesting data is one thing, but understanding these data is quite another" (p. 3342). The propagation and the success of polluted information are socio-technical phenomena; as such, the technical and social domains should be integrated.

5.2. JUGGLING DIVERGENT NEEDS

The analysis of the main characteristics and roles of providers, supporters, and receivers, and of how they build their identities and systems of beliefs through their different drifting in and out medical misinformation, shed light on core online socialization mechanisms informing the propagation and success of some dangerous health-related beliefs, including those we experienced during the pandemic. In order to disrupt – and possibly prevent – potentially harmful misinformation through better designed, framed, and targeted science-based information and public health-related communication, however, equally important is the identification of the prevalent and convergent narrative frames, and the epistemological mechanisms at the basis of the misinformation witnessed. We have seen, for instance, that even if the frequency, duration, and intensity of participation in online discussions can vary, and there is no clear socio-cultural homogeneity, there are shared themes and narratives that, besides facilitating socialization with what are perceived as like-minded people, are also useful to engage larger audiences. The different logics and the different spheres of discourse and practice often involved in science-based and non-science based approaches (Barcan, 2015) need to be unpacked in order to create a bridge to effectively communicate with those drifting more and more into misinformation, improving if not the frequency or duration and least the intensity and quality of their "good information" exposure. As (all) people's perceptions of social groups are based on stereotypes and there is a tendency to personalize groups as collective agents (Biddlestone et al., 2020), also stereotypes on groups endorsing alternative or conspiratorial thinking often determine judgments about social groups as a whole, regardless of the variety of actors associated with those groups.

As such, any individual or public intervention aiming at disrupting or preventing medical misinformation cannot avoid to engage with the puzzle of how to reconcile the (diverse) needs and the rights of some with the interests of society at large. After all, in the context of public health, striving for a difficult balance between individual rights and public interest, fairness, and efficacy, has a long (and at times ethically controversial) history, and only in the more extreme cases individual agency can be override to reduce, for instance, the risk of a disease spreading to the rest of the community (Fahlquist, 2019) – something that cannot be justified in the overwhelming majority of the online conversations observed. In most cases, interfering top-down in the drift equilibria to give people relatively more "good information" exposure by limiting the publication or dissemination of misinformation would be possible only by middling with free speech protection and the individual right to self-expression – something that cannot be welcomed in democratic societies. Similarly, top-down interventions trying to control the flow of information online would stir us toward a "paternal internet" model (O'Hara and Hall, 2018; Smart et al., 2019) – again not a good solution if we want to maintain commitment to the free and libertarian nature of cyberspace, and to net neutrality. This is why – as we will soon discuss – alternative solutions are needed, with media, the private sector, and researchers themselves being in a very important position to contribute to the mitigation of harms.

Top-down solutions are also hindered by the fact that there is a core element of individual risk acceptance, as opposed to societal risk management and control (Beck, 1992; Martin & Johnson, 2001; Figuié, 2014) – a tension that cannot elude to reopen and further the brief parenthesis started in Section 1.3 on moral responsibility (Fahlquist, 2019) as linked to social harms (Hillyard and Tombs, 2008). Individual moral responsibility in health choices with repercussions for others (as in the case of vaccine refusal) has been long debated (with recent scholarship arguing that individuals who, for instance, opt out of vaccination are morally responsible for resultant harms to others – see, for instance, Jamrozik et al., 2016; Giubilini et al., 2018), and it is likely that this issue will soon be further theorized with reference to pandemic-specific behaviors (such as antimasks). Issues of collective moral responsibility (which address widespread harms associated with the actions of groups) in this context, however, have been less debated, not only because the notion itself of collective moral responsibility is much more contested (Held, 1970; Dan-Cohen, 1986; Hayward, 2006), but probably also because, in the online networks analyzed, individuals tend to cluster in collectives that are transient and situational, and not stable enough to be considered moral agents in their own right.

In the context of medical misinformation during the pandemic, however, issues of moral responsibility do not affect only those who are actively engaged as promoters and supporters online, but they also affect a broader intermingled system made up – among others – by a number of collective and individual moral agents including online intermediaries, traditional media outlets, and bad communicators; and this system is worsened by regulatory loopholes. This study does not have the pre-tension to untangle this maze, but it is nonetheless important to recognize the complexity of the matter, and that any discussion of moral responsibility or harm prevention and minimization cannot escape an analysis of the broader infrastructural and societal context enabling and leading individual behaviors.

5.3. RECOGNIZING THE MAZE

Among the regulatory loopholes facilitating medical misinformation, there is one in particular whose existence was at the very core of some of the practices observed in this study. Indeed, in the discourses analyzed, too often providers and supporters were able to play with the confusion and ambiguities that the general public has around what is "alternative medicine" – a confusion long fostered in Italy by traditional media (Lavorgna and

Di Ronco, 2018) – presenting both themselves and their unplausible health approaches as dignified by belonging to the big house of CAMs. This equivocation is indeed linked to the ambiguities around the definition of CAMs itself, and of CAM practitioners. As mentioned in the introductory chapter, in Italy as in many other western countries health care underwritten by the state is (supposed to be) based on science-based medicine – or "orthodox" medicine as this is sometimes called by CAM researchers, who stress its biomedical dominance and the focus on drugs and surgery (Saks, 2015). Conversely, CAM is used as a sort of umbrella term covering a broad range of therapies and approaches that generally are not supported by the state; what is included under the CAM umbrella is not a stable list, but a shifting one depending on different societies and jurisdictions (Saks, 2015). In Italy, filling a legislative void, in 2002 the National Federation for the Orders of Doctors and Dentist formally recognized as non-conventional medicine only nine disciplines (acupuncture, phytotherapy, homeopathy, traditional Chinese medicine, anthroposophical medicine, Ayurveda, homotossicology, osteopathy, and chiropractic). These disciplines can complement, and not substitute, science-based medicine and are under the competence and responsibility of doctors, dentists, veterinaries, or pharmacists; other providers cannot legally offer diagnosis, preventive treatments, and cures (FNOMCeO, 2002). However, over the years this system proved dangerously ineffective in countering harmful forms of alternative health approaches, which have been prospering in the country (Lavorgna and Di Ronco, 2017; D'Amato, 2019).

Also, in recognized forms of CAMs, whether someone is "professional" or not remains a source of debate, as the word professional can be used both for those subject to formal statutory regulatory processes and ethical codes, and for those who simply have a specific level of competence in a designated activity (McHale, 2015). Since 2013, some Italian provinces have lists of legally recognized providers of acupuncture, phytotherapy, and homeopathy (54/CSR, February 7, 2013) – hence providing only a partial regulation of a much wider issue. There are ongoing debates on the necessity or even the opportunity to regulate CAMs: some CAM practitioners think that more stringent regulations might confer them professional legitimacy and status and, as such, welcome the idea of regulatory interventions; others are afraid to be subject to too many constraints, and argue that existing civil and criminal law remedies are already enough to make practitioners accountable if or when harms arise (McHale, 2015). Some of those critical toward CAMs oppose regulatory interventions for the very same reason that they are afraid these interventions would confer legitimacy and status to some practitioners; others welcome more stringent regulations to safeguard the public (Iyioha, 2015).

Considering how the providers and supporters encountered in this study exploit the ambiguities allowed by current regulatory loopholes, and the fact that the societal needs they are filling are not going to disappear anytime soon, the lack of a stricter regulatory intervention is increasingly resembling an ostrich policy. In medical contexts, it is not unusual for the state to abrogate responsibility (Devaney and Holm, 2018); but if responsibility is not to be framed (only) as an individual issue but as a societal issue, and we recognize that vulnerability is universal and constant and differences among people depend on the different distribution of dependency, privilege, and resilience within our society (Fineman, 2013), further state intervention and monitoring should be welcomed (Garland and Travis, 2020) also in the CAM arena.

Among the main actors that are part of the complex and intermingled system fostering medical misinformation mentioned above, are online intermediaries. Especially social media companies have been under the spotlight in the pandemic for being a vessel of misinformation. Despite the declared efforts and the announces that they were expanding their policies around COVID-19-related misinformation – such as removing millions of individual posts presenting false claims about cures, treatments, and the vaccines while prioritizing trusted sources offering "prompts" on their platforms to direct users toward public health agencies – it is clear that these methods to curb polluted information are not as effective as hoped. The underlying problem is that social media are not designed with issues such as the polluted information (or, more generally, social harms) in mind. However, we should not forget that cyberspace is a built environment, shaped by its architects (ranging from the software designers to the site administrators); changes in its architecture have direct effects in people's interactions (Donath, 1996; Floridi, 1996), making conversations more or less spontaneous, affecting trust and social pressures, and indirectly affecting the spread of (mis)information. The ways in which architectural changes can evolve and be implemented are not easy to determine and assess. Nonetheless, it is not unthinkable that it their evolution social media companies (with the right incentives) could develop in a way that architecturally makes misinformation and, more generally, polluted information more difficult to thrive – certainly an issue deserving more attention in the near future.

Also traditional media outlets proved problematic as potential enablers of misinformation. As mentioned in Section 1.2, in Italy (as in other countries) many traditional media – even those that would commonly be considered as trustworthy sources of information – too often failed appropriate reporting of science-based pandemic-related information, increasing information pollution (Marino and Serani, 2020), and confirming their inadequacy in discerning – and helping the public to discern – among good and misinformation in health-related matters (Lavorgna and Di Ronco, 2018). The relationship between science, its communication, science–media interactions, and the responsibilities for acts of communications and acts of silence (as they both open up spaces of interpretation) is a very complex one. At the heart of it, are the conundrum on when is best to engage with the general public about an emerging field of science, as badly timed communication might create unfounded hopes or even fears, and the use of responsible language (Nerlich and McLeod, 2016). Arguably there have been mistakes in the communicative strategies around COVID-19 and, at the time of the completion of this book, around vaccination strategies, and these mistakes exceed media outlets' responsibilities. Too often, communication of scientific expertise was not entrusted to professional science communicators, but left to scientists and doctors themselves. While these categories have certainly an important role in the science–society relationships (Peters, 2014), they are not always well versed in dealing with the logic of mass media, with the consequence that too often scientific expertise entered general public debates and even the realm of policymaking in a troubling way.

As a repercussion, some (possibly well-intentioned) individual agents inadvertently ended up fostering social harms in the pandemic. We have seen in Section 3.3, for instance, how "celebrity scientists" entered the public debate, often showing divisive voices. Visible, or public, scientists are nothing new in modern science, especially in the aftermath of the social transformations of late modernity and the increasingly pervasive use of cyberspace that redefined and multiplied spaces for science communication (Bucchi and Trench, 2014). In Italy, during the pandemic, some scientists and doctors got a lot of public visibility via social media, a visibility at times further amplified through their participation in television programs. In popular discourses, these scientists have been associated with discourses of truth, reason, rationality, and progress, as if their public images have an epistemological dimension (Joseph and Sullivan, 1975; Fahy and Lewenstein, 2014), even when unfortunately the "celebrity status" acquired enabled them to comment also on areas outside their realm of expertise, providing inaccurate information to their "believers" while further hindering trust on them by those more skeptic.

Additionally, it was not uncommon to see active in cyberspace online users and scientists improvised debunkers trying to convince their audiences of the validity of certain data or certain science-based approaches. Unfortunately, most scientists and researchers are not trained to promote community-level science literacy, and are not prepared to engage (also on social media) with the general public (Sharon and Baram-Tsabari, 2020). As such, if providers and supporters proficiently managed to build a convenient "us vs them" narrative, such narrative was only reinforced by some of these bad communicators furthering forms of "cybersanctioning" such ridiculing, shaming, and stigmatizing as gullible those believing certain (mis) information. All these methods, indeed, assume that there is a shared system of beliefs to which to conform: teasing and mocking are supposedly used as incentives to change behavior, with the idea that fear of being ridiculed might be a motivator to conform; also shame and stigmatization can be used as a method of social control by provoking guilt or embarrassment (Thompson and Gibbs, 2017). In lack of this shared system (and we have seen that the biological implausibility or the conspiracist ideation behind certain health-related approaches are no longer fringe beliefs), however, these methods lose their status of informal social control mechanisms, and rather become forms of cyberharassment.

Furthermore, even when debunking was not confrontational but only factual, some problems remain: first, fact-checking is a scarce resource (Brennen et al., 2020), and it is unpractical to think to be able to respond effectively to countless plainly wrong or counterinformative claims. Even more importantly, debunking relies on the questionable assumptions that certain alternative theories are statements about facts, and that their "followers," by believing in them, are deviant as they deviate from positive knowledge (Hristov, 2019, p. 92). These assumptions, however, have been proved wrong: conspiratorial thinking, for instance, does not have a stable form (unlike factual statements), and certain systems of beliefs are often perceived only half-seriously as entertainment or curiosity; they seduce their readers in a subliminal way that escapes rational calculation (Hristov, 2019; Landrum and Olshansky, 2019). Besides having an epistemological incompatibility, there can also be a misalignment of goals between, for instance, intuitive spiritual or healing practices and science-based medicine: to borrow Barcan's (2015) words, *"they are fundamentally different spheres of discourse and practice, animated by different logics. Healing essentially means reconciliation, which may occur on a physical, mental, emotional, social or spiritual plane, and may not always involve the eradication of the disease. Indeed, in some cases even death itself – a peaceful, reconciled death – may be understood as a form of healing, in stark contrast to the triumphalist aspirations typifying the biomedical paradigm"* (p. 229).

As such, all the communicative strategies listed so far tend to be ineffective and even counterproductive, and can unintentionally stimulate antiscientific thinking by entering an endless duel with it. There is research on mistrust in science that can offer important food for thought: research on vaccine hesitancy or refusal, for example, suggests that, as individual epistemologies drive some health-related decisions and communal embeddedness validate them, using the same communicative characteristics that are successful in antivax communities – rather than fighting them – can be more effective (Duchsherer et al., 2020). For instance, anecdotes and personal examples can be more effective than the simple delivery of statistical information; empathy-driven and tailored patient-provider dialogues are to be preferred to impersonal public messaging (Baron and Berinsky, 2019; Prot and Anderson 2019; Duchsherer et al., 2020). As ideology and cultural worldview play an important role in science denial, and cultural cognition affects also whom people believe (individuals are more likely to view an expert as credible and trustworthy if they believe that the expert share their cultural values, see Kahan et al., 2010), it is important to present information in a way that can align with people's cultural values and ideologies, rather than threatening them, and to involve a diverse set of experts in scientific communication, so to improve chances to have at least one expert perceived as credible by people with different worldviews (Sherman and Cohen, 2006; Kahan et al., 2010; Prot and Anderson 2019).

Furthermore, we know that how experts communicate risks and benefits in the context of vaccination matters, as it impacts public trust – which is not a mean but rather should be seen as the result of ethically justified public health activities. In this context, treating certain people's concerns as irrational or overly emotional is useless and rather counterproductive, as certain emotions are and should be part of a discussion on the moral acceptability of risk (Fahlquist, 2019, p. 125). Of course, as Fahlquist herself clarifies, insisting that people's concerns should be taken seriously does not imply a relativistic view or the equation of facts, opinions, and values: rather, taking these concerns seriously allows to establish an attentive dialogue, which is needed to maintain, build, or restore public trust, and consequently public health. Hence, public discourses opposing the utilitarian goals of public health and claims of individual liberty, in a sort of false dichotomy of Reason vs Emotion (Fahlquist, 2019), should be avoided.

Kreko (2020) conceptualized existing interventions aimed to counter conspiracy theories – but his approach can be adapted also to conceptualize interventions toward polluted information – by putting them on a two-dimensional matrix built across a temporal dimension (from prevention to harm reduction) and a target dimension (depending on whether the intervention targets the messenger/source of the information or its recipients). The matrix offers four possible options: (1) pre-emptive strike (the intervention takes place before the spread of the message and targets the source); (2) immunization (it takes place before the dissemination but targets the recipient); (3) striking back (it takes place after the message was spread and targets the source); and (4) healing (it takes place after the dissemination but targets the recipient). So far, interventions targeting polluted information have not taken place in a coordinated way. Some, especially those technology-focused led by online intermediaries, have been targeting the source; as discussed above, in lack of more profound architectural interventions these approaches are proving relatively ineffective, and can potentially create serious tensions against individual rights. Debunking activities have been targeting the recipients, but too often in a very ineffective and counterproductive way, increasing polarization and facilitating displacement toward more protected social media. As is the case with other online harms, there is no single best strategy for the control or prevention of polluted information and medical misinformation (Brennen et al., 2020): in order for proper immunization and healing to occur, a sustained, concerted, and multilayered effort between a wide range of institutions, individual actors, and technology is therefore needed. A very challenging task indeed, but one we cannot evade.

REFERENCES

Abbott, A. 2001. *Chaos of Disciplines*, Chicago, IL, University of Chicago Press.

Adhanom Ghebreyesus, T. 2020. *WHO Director General Speech, Munich Security Conference*, February 15. Available at: https://www.who.int/dg/speeches/detail/munich-security-conference

Agrafiotis, I., Bada, M., Cornish, P., Creese, S., Goldsmith, M., Ignatuschtschenko, E., Roberts, T. and Upton, D. 2016. *Cyber Harm: Concepts, Taxonomy and Measurement*, Working Paper No. 2016-23, Saïd Business School, Oxford, UK.

Agrafiotis, I., Nurse, J.R.C., Goldsmith, M., Creese, S. and Upton, D. 2018. A taxonomy of cyber-harms: Defining the impacts of cyber-attacks and understanding how they propagate, *Journal of Cybersecurity*, 4(1).

Akers, R. 2009. *Social Learning and Social Structure: A General Theory of Crime and Deviance*, New Brunswick, NJ, Transaction.

Alaszewski, A. 2015. Anthropology and risk: insights into uncertainty, danger and blame from other cultures – a review essay, *Health, Risks and Society*, 17(3–4), 205–225.

Alich, A. 2015. Shamanism and safety. Ancient practices and modern issues. In *Routledge Handbook of Complementary and Alternative Medicine. Perspectives from Social Science and Law*, Eds N.K. Gale and J.V. McHale, London, Routledge.

Allcott, H. and Gentzkow, M. 2017. Social media and fake news in the 2016 elections, *Journal of Economic Perspectives*, 31(2), 211–236.

Amarasingam, A. and Argentino, M.A. 2020. The QAnon conspiracy theory: a security threat in the making?, *CTC Sentinel*, 13(7), 37–44.

Androutsopoulos, J. 2008. Potential and limitations of discourse-centred online ethnography, *Language@Internet*, 5(9), 1–20.

Artime, O., D'Andrea, V., Gallotti, R., Sacco, P.L. and De Domenico, M. 2020. Effectiveness of dismantling strategies on moderated vs unmoderated online social platforms. arXiv:2004.14879v1 [physics.soc-ph]

Aupers, S. 2020. Decoding mass media/encoding conspiracy theory. In *Routledge Handbook of Conspiracy Theories*, Eds M. Butter and P. Knight, London, Routledge.

Bangerter, A., Wagner-Egger, P. and Delouvee, S. 2020. How conspiracy theories spread. In *Routledge Handbook of Conspiracy Theories*, Eds M. Butter and P. Knight, London, Routledge.

Barcan, R. 2015. Intuitive spiritual medicine. Negotiating incommensurability. In *Routledge Handbook of Complementary and Alternative Medicine. Perspectives from Social Science and Law*, Eds N.K. Gale and J.V. McHale, London, Routledge.

Baron, R.J. and Berinsky, A.J. 2019. Mistrust in science – a threat to the patient-physician relationship, *The New England Journal of Medicine*, 381(2), 182–185.

Basham, L. 2001. Living with the conspiracy, *The Philosophical Forum*, 32(3), 256–280.

Beck, U. 1992. *Risk Society: Towards a New Modernity*, London, Sage.

Berendt, B., Gandon, F., Halford, S., Hall, W., Hendler, J., Kindr-Kurlanda, K., Ntoutsi, E. and Staab, S. 2020. *Web Futures: Inclusive, Intelligent, Sustainable. The 2020 Manifesto for Web Science*. Available at: https://www.webscience.org/wp-content/uploads/sites/117/2020/07/main.pdf

Blevins, K.R. and Holt, T.J. 2009. Examining the virtual subculture of Johns, *Journal of Contemporary Ethnography*, 38(5), 619–648.

Biddlestone, M., Cichocka, A., Zezeli, I. and Bilewicz, M. 2020. In *Routledge Handbook of Conspiracy Theories*, Eds M. Butter and P. Knight, London, Routledge.

Boaz, D. 2008. *The Politics of Freedom: Taking on the Left, the Right and Threats to Our Liberties*, Washington, DC, Cato Institute.

Boyle, J. 1996. *Shamans, Software, and Spleens: Law and the Construction of the Information Society*, Cambridge, MA, Harvard University Press.

Braun, V., Clarke, V., Hayfield, N. and Terry, G. 2019. Thematic analysis. In *Handbook of Research Methods in Health Social Sciences*, Ed. P. Liamputtong, Singapore, Springer.

References

Brennen, J.S., Simon, F., Howard, P.N. and Nielsen, R.K. 2020. *Types, Sources and Claims of COVID-19 Disinformation*, Oxford, Reuters Institute.

Brewer, M.B. 2007. The social psychology of intergroup relations: social categorization, ingroup bias, and outgroup prejudice. In *Social Psychology: Handbook of Basic Principles*, Eds A.W. Kruglanski and E.T. Higgins, New York, NY, Guilford Press.

Bricken, M. 1991. *Virtual Worlds: No Interface to Design*. Technical Report No. R-90-2. Human Interface Technology Laboratory, University of Washington, Seattle.

Broniatowski, D.A., Jamison, A.M., Qi, S., AlKulaib, L., Chen, T., Benton, A., Quinn, S.A. and Dredze, M. 2018. Weaponized health communication: twitter bots and Russian trolls amplify the vaccine debate, *American Journal of Public Health*, 108(10), 1378–1384.

Brooker, P., Dutton, W. and Greiffenhagen, C. 2017. What would Wittgenstein say about social media?, *Qualitative Research*, 17(6), 610–626.

Brown, P. 2020. Studying COVID-19 in light of critical approaches to risk and uncertainty: research pathways, conceptual tools, and some magic from Mary Douglas, *Health Risk and Society*, 22(1), 1–14.

Bruns, A. 2008. *Blogs, Wikipedia, Second Life and Beyond: From Production to Produsage*, New York, NY, Peter Lang.

BSA. 2017. *Ethics Guidelines and Collated Resources for Digital Research: Statement of Ethical Practice Annex*, Durham, British Sociological Association. Available at: https://www.britsoc.co.uk/media/24309/bsa_statement_of_ethical_practice_annexe.pdf

Bucchi, M. and Trench, B. 2014. Science communication research. Themes and challenges. In *Routledge Handbook of Public Communication of Science and Technology*, Eds M. Bucchi and B. Trench, London, Routledge.

Camus, A. 1947/2004. *The Plague*, New York, NY, Everyman's Library.

Cassidy, A. 2014. Commutating the social sciences. A specific challenge? In *Routledge Handbook of Public Communication of Science and Technology*, Eds M. Bucchi and B. Trench, London, Routledge.

Cattaneo, E. and Corbellini, G. 2014. Taking a stand against pseudoscience, *Nature*, 510, 333–335.

Chung, J.E. 2014. Social networking in online support groups for health: how online social networking benefits patients, *Journal of Health Communications*, 19(6), 639–659.

City of London Police. 2020. *Man Charged with Making and Selling Fake COVID-19 Treatment Kits.* Available at: http://news.cityoflondon.police.uk/r/1332/man_charged_with_making_and_selling_fake_covid-19

Cloatre, E. 2019. Traditional medicines, law, and the (dis)ordering of temporalities. In *Law and Time*, Eds S.M. Beynon-Jones and E. Grabham, London, Routledge.

Coday, D. 2006. An introduction to the philosophical debate about conspiracy theories. In *Conspiracy Theories. The Philosophical Debate*, Ed. D. Coday, London, Routledge.

Collins, H. and Evans, R. 2008. *Rethinking Expertise*, Chicago, IL, University of Chicago Press.

Conrad, P., Bandini, J. and Vasquez, A. 2016. Illness and the Internet: from private to public experience, *Health: An Interdisciplinary Journal for the Social Study of Health, Illness and Medicine*, 20(1), 22–32.

Copes, H. and Ragland, J. 2016. Considering the implicit meaning in photographs in narrative criminology, *Crime, Media, Culture*, 12(2), 271.

Copes, H., Hochstetler, A. and Ragland, J. 2019. The stories in images: the value of the visual for narrative criminology. In *The Emerald Handbook for Narrative Criminology*, Eds J. Fleetwood, L. Presser, S. Sandberg and T. Ugelvik, Bingley, Emerald.

CPS. 2020. *"Coronavirus Coughs" At Key Workers Will Be Charged as Assault, CPS Warns* Available at: https://www.cps.gov.uk/cps/news/coronavirus-coughs-key-workers-will-be-charged-assault-cps-warns

Cosentino, G. 2020. *Social Media and the Post-Truth World Order: The Global Dynamics of Disinformation*, London, Palgrave Macmillan.

D'Amato, I. 2019. Dossier Hamer: the role of investigative journalism in exposing pseudomedicine. In *Medical Misinformation and Social Harm in Non-Science-Based Health Practices: A Multidisciplinary Perspective*, Eds A. Lavorgna and A. Di Ronco, London, Routledge.

Dan-Cohen, M. 1986. *Rights, Persons, and Organizations*, Berkeley, CA, University of California Press.

Davies, P., Francis, P. and Greer, C. 2017. *Victims, Crime & Society*, London, Sage.

de Certeau, M. 1984. *The Practice of Everyday Life*, Berkeley, CA, University of California Press.

References

Del Vicario, M., Bessi, A., Zollo, F., Petroni, F., Scala, A., Caldarelli, G., Stanley, E. and Quattrociocchi, W. 2016. The spreading of misinformation online. *Proceedings of the National Academy of Sciences of the United States of America*, 113(3), 554–559.

Devaney, S. and Holm, S. 2018. The transmutation of deference in medicine: an ethico-legal perspective, *Medical Law Review*, 202, 224.

Di Ronco, A. and Allen-Robertson, J. 2019. Activism against medicine on social media: untangling the #novax protest in Italy on Twitter. In *Medical Misinformation and Social Harm in Non-Science-Based Health Practices: A Multidisciplinary Perspective*, Eds A. Lavorgna and A. Di Ronco, London, Routledge.

Donath, J. 1996. Identity and deception in the virtual community. In *Communities in Cyberspace*, Eds P. Kollock and M. Smith, London, Routledge.

Donath, J. 2014. *The Social Machine. Design for Living Online*, Cambridge, MA, The MIT Press.

Donovan, J. 2020. Social-media companies must flatten the curve of misinformation, *Nature*. doi:10.1038/d41586-020-01107-z. Availble at: https://www.nature.com/articles/d41586-020-01107-z.

Douglas, K.M., Cichocka, A. and Sutton, R.M. 2020. Motivations, emotions and belief in conspiracy theories. In *Routledge Handbook of Conspiracy Theories*, Eds M. Butter and P. Knight, London, Routledge.

Douglas, M. 1992. *Risk and Blame: Essay in Cultural Theory*, London, Routledge.

Duchsherer, A., Jason, M., Platt, C.A. and Majdik, Z.P. 2020. Immunized against science: narrative community building among vaccine refusing/hesitant parents. *Public Understanding of Science* (online first).

Ernst, E. 2019. *Alternative Medicine*, Cham, Copernicus.

Fahlquist, J.N. 2019. *Moral Responsibility and Risk in Society. Examples from Emerging Technologies, Public Health and the Environment*, London, Routledge.

Fahy, D. and Lewenstein, B.V. 2014. Scientists in popular culture. The making of celebrities. In *Routledge Handbook of Public Communication of Science and Technology*, Eds M. Bucchi and B. Trench, London, Routledge.

Feinberg, J. 1984. *Harm to Others – The Moral Limits of the Criminal Law*, New York, NY, Oxford University Press.

Ferguson, T. 1997. Health care in cyberspace: patients lead a revolution, *The Futurist*, 61(6), 29–33.

Ferrell, J. 1999. Cultural criminology, *Annual Review of Sociology*, 25, 395–418.

Ferrell, J. and Hamm, M. 1998. True confessions: crime, deviance and the field research. In *Ethnography on the Edge*, Eds J. Ferrell and M. Hamm, Boston, MA, Northeastern University Press.

Ferrell, J., Haywards, K. and Young, J. 2008. *Cultural Criminology: An Invitation*, London, Sage.

Figuié, M. 2014. Towards a global governance of risks: international health organisations and the surveillance of emerging infectious diseases, *Journal of Risk Research*, 17(4), 469–483.

Fineman, M. 2013. *The Vulnerable Subject: Anchoring Equality in the Human Condition*, Princeton, NJ, Princeton University Press.

Fischer, J.M. and Ravizza, M. 1998. *Responsibility and Control: A Theory of Moral Responsibility*, Cambridge, Cambridge University Press.

Floridi, L. 1996. Brave.Net.World: the Internet as a disinformation superhighway?, *The Electronic Library*, 14(6), 509–514.

FNOMCeO. 2002. *Linee guida della federazione nazionale degli ordini dei medici chirurghi e degli odontoiatri su medicine e pratiche non convenzionali.* Available at: http://www.amnco.it/server/Delibera_Terni02_MNC.pdf

Forsyth, D.R. 2019. *Group Dynamics*, 7th ed., Andover, Cengage.

Foucault, M. 1988. *Technologies of the Self: A Seminar with Michel Foucault*, Amherst, MA, University of Massachusetts Press.

Foucault, M. 2001. *Fearless Speech*, Los Angeles, CA, Semiotext(e).

French, M., Mykhalovskiy, E. and Lamothe, C. 2018. Epidemics, pandemics, and outbreaks. In *The Cambridge Handbook of Social Problems*, Ed. J. Trevino, Cambridge, Cambridge University Press.

Fuchs, C. 2019. What is critical digital social research? Five reflections on the study of digital society, *Journal of Digital Social Research*, 1(1), 10–16.

Fuchs, C., Hofkirchner, W., Schafranek, M., Raffl, C., Sandoval, M. and Bichler, R. 2010. Theoretical foundations of the Web: cognition, communication, and co operation. Towards an understanding of Web 1.0, 2.0, 3.0, *Future Internet*, 2, 41–59.

Fullwood, C., Chadwick, D., Keep, M., Attrill-Smith, A., Asbury, T. and Kirwan, G. 2019. Lurking towards empowerment: explaining propensity to engage with online health support groups and its association with positive outcomes, *Computers in Human Behaviours*, 90, 131–140.

Garland, F. and Travis, M. 2020. Making the state responsible: intersex embodiment, medical jurisdiction and state responsibility, *Journal of Law and Society*, 47(2), 298–324.

Gazzola, E. 2019. Quantum physics and the modern trends in pseudoscience. In *Medical Misinformation and Social Harm in Non-Science-Based Health Practices: A Multidisciplinary Perspective*, Eds A. Lavorgna and A. Di Ronco, London, Routledge.

Geertz, C. 1973. *The Interpretation of Cultures*, New York, NY, Basic Books.

Gentilviso, C. and Aikat, D. 2019. Embracing the visual, verbal, and viral media: how post-millennial consumption habits are reshaping the news. In *Mediated Millennials*, Eds J. Schulz, L. Robinson, A. Khilnani, J. Baldwin, H. Pait, A.A. Williams, J. Davis and G. Ignatow, Bingley, Emerald Publishing.

Gergen, K. and Gergen, M. 1983. Narratives of the self. In *Studies in Social Identity*, Eds T. Sarbin and K. Scheibe, New York, NY, Praeger.

Giles, D., Stommel, W., Paulus, T., Lester, J. and Reed, D. 2015. Microanalysis of online data: The methodological development of "digital CA", *Discourse, Context and Media*, 7(3), 45–51.

Giubilini, A., Douglas, T. and Savulescu, J. 2018. The moral obligation to be vaccinated: utilitarianism, contractualism, and collective easy rescue, *Medicine, Health Care and Philosophy*, 21, 547–560.

Godlee, F. 2011. Wakefield's article linking MMR vaccine and autism was fraudulent. *Editorial, The British Medical Journal*, 342, c7452.

Goffman, E. 1959. *The Presentation of Self in Everyday Life*, New York, NY, Doubleday.

Goffman, E. 1963. *Stigma: Notes on the Management of Spoiled Identity*, New York, NY, Touchstone.

Goffman, E. 1983. The interaction order: American Sociological Association, 1982 presidential address. *American Sociological Review*, 48(1), 1–17.

Goldberg, R.A. 2008. *Enemies Within: The Culture of Conspiracy in Modern America*, New Haven, CT, Yale University Press.

Goldman, A. and O'Connor, C. 2019. Social epistemology. In *The Stanford Encyclopedia of Philosophy*, Ed. E.N. Zalta.

Goldsmith, A. and Brewer, R. 2015. Digital drift and the criminal interaction order, *Theoretical Criminology*, 19(1), 112–130.

Grabosky, P.N., Smith, R.G. and Wright, P. 1998. Crime in the digital age. In *Controlling Telecommunications and Cyberspace Illegalities*, New Brunswick, NJ, Transaction Publishers.

Harabman, J. and Aupers, S. 2014. Contesting epistemic authority: Conspiracy theories on the boundaries of science, *Public Understanding of Science*, 24(4), 466–480.

Haines, H.H. 1981. The deviant subject: David Matza's sociology of deviance, *Mid-American Review of Sociology*, 6(1), 51–69.

Halford, S., Pope, C. and Weal, M. 2013. Digital futures? Sociological challenges and opportunities in the emergent Semantic Web, *Sociology*, 47(1), 173–189.

Halford, S., Weal, M., Tinati, R., Carr, L. and Pope, C. 2018. Understanding the production and circulation of social media data: towards methodological principles and praxis, *New Media & Society*, 20(9), 3341–3358.

Hayward, C.R. 2006. On power and responsibility, *Political Studies Review*, 4, 156–163.

Hayward, K. 2004. *City Limits: Crime, Consumer Culture and the Urban Experience*, London, Glasshouse Press.

Hayward, K.J. and Young, J. 2004. Cultural criminology: Some notes on the script, *Theoretical Criminology*, 8(3), 259–273.

Held, V. 1970. Can a random collective be morally responsible?, *Journal of Philosophy*, 6, 471–481.

Herbert, V. 1986. Unproven (questionable) dietary and nutritional methods in cancer prevention and treatment, *Cancer*, 58(S8), 1930–1941.

Hillyard, P., Pantazis, C., Tombs, S. and Gordon, D. Eds 2004. *Beyond Criminology: Taking Crime Seriously*, London, Pluto Press.

Hillyard, P. and Tombs, S. 2008. Beyond criminology?. In *Criminal Obsessions: Why Harm Matters More Than Crime*, Eds D. Dorling, D. Gordon, P. Hillyard, C. Pantazis, S. Pemberton and S. Tombs, 2nd ed., London, Centre for Crime and Justice Studies.

References

Hogg, M.A. 2016. Social identity theory. In *Understanding Peace and Conflict through Social Identity Theory*, Eds S. McKeown, R. Haji and N. Ferguson, Cham, Springer.

Holt, T.J., Brewer, R. and Goldsmith, A. 2019. Digital drift and the "sense of injustice": counter-productive policing of youth cybercrime, *Deviant Behavior*, 40(9), 1144–1156.

Hotez, P. 2019. America and Europe's new normal: the return of vaccine-preventable diseases, *Nature Pediatric Research*, 85, 912–914.

Housley, W., Webb, H., Edwards, A., Procter, R. and Jirotka, M. 2017. Digitizing sacks? Approaching social media as data, *Qualitative Research*, 17(6), 627–644.

Howard, W.J. 2017. Punishment as moral fortification, *Law and Philosophy*, 36, 45–75.

Hristov, T. 2019. *Impossible Knowledge: Conspiracy Theories, Power and Truth*, London, Routledge.

Imhoff, R. and Lamberty, P. 2020. Conspiracy beliefs as psycho-political reactions to perceived power. In *Routledge Handbook of Conspiracy Theories*, Eds M. Butter and P. Knight, London, Routledge.

ImparareSicuri. 2020. Osservatorio civico sulla sicurezza a scuola. Available at: https://www.cittadinanzattiva.it/files/primo_piano/scuola/rapporto-scuola-xvii/ABSTRACT_XVII_Sicurezza.pdf

ISTAT. 2020. Spazi in casa e disponibilita' di computer per bambini e ragazzi. Available at: https://www.istat.it/it/files/2020/04/Spazi-casa-disponibilita-computer-ragazzi.pdf

Iyioha, I.O. 2015. The harm principle and liability for CAM practice. A comparative analysis of Canadian and United States health freedom laws. In *Routledge Handbook of Complementary and Alternative Medicine. Perspectives from Social Science and Law*, Eds N.K. Gale and J.V. McHale, London, Routledge.

Jamrozik, E., Handfield, T. and Selgelid, M.J. 2016. Victims, vectors and villains: are those who opt out of vaccination morally responsible for the deaths of others?, *Journal of Medical Ethics*, 42, 762–768.

Johnson, N.F., Velásquez, N. and Restrepo, N.J. 2020. The online competition between pro- and anti-vaccination views, *Nature*, 582, 230–233.

Joseph, B.D. and Sullivan, T.A. 1975. Sociology of science, *Annual Review of Sociology*, 1(1), 203–222.

Jowett, A. 2015. A case for using online discussion forums in critical psychological research, *Qualitative Research in Psychology*, 12(3), 287–297.

Kahan, D.M., Braman, D., Cohen, G., Slovic, P. and Gastil, J. 2010. Who fears the HPV vaccine, who doesn't, and why: an experimental study of the mechanisms of cultural cognition, *Law and Human Behavior*, 34(6), 501–516.

Kaptchuk, T.J. and Eisenberg, D.M. 1998. The persuasive appeal of alternative medicine, *Annals of Internal Medicine*, 129(12), 1061–1065.

Katz, J. 1988. *Seductions of Crime: Moral and Sensual Attractions in Doing Evil*, New York, NY, Basic Books.

Keeley, B.L. 1999. Of conspiracy theories. *Journal of Philosophy*, XCVI(3), 109–126.

Kennedy, P.J. and Prat, A. 2019. Where do people get their news?, *Economic Policy*, 34(97), 5–47.

Khamis, S., Lawrence, A. and Raymond, W. 2016. Self-branding, "micro-celebrity" and the rise of social media influencers, *Celebrity Studies*, 8(2), 191–208.

Klawitter, E. and Hargittai, E. 2018. "I went home to Google": how user assess the credibility of online health information. In *eHealth: Current Evidence, Promises, Perils and Future Directions*, Eds T.M. Hale, W.Y.S. Chou, S.R. Cotton and A. Khilnani, Bingley, Emerald.

Klein, O. and Nera, K. 2020. Social psychology of conspiracy theories. In *Routledge Handbook of Conspiracy Theories*, Eds M. Butter and P. Knight, London, Routledge.

Koenig, H.G., Idler, E., Kasl, S., Hays, J.C., George, L.K., Musick, M., Larson, D.B., Collins, T.R. and Benson, H. 1999. Religion, spirituality, and medicine: a rebuttal to skeptics, *International Journal of Psychiatry in Medicine*, 29(2), 123–131.

Konnikova, M. 2016. Mind games: how con artists get the better of you, *New Scientist*, January 20. Available at: https://www.newscientist.com/article/2073748-mind-games-how-con-artists-get-the-better-of-you/.

Kozinets, R.V. 2010. *Netnography: Doing Ethnographic Research Online*, London, Sage.

Krause, N.M., Brossard, D., Scheufele, D.A., Xenos, M.A. and Franke, K. 2019. Trends – Americans' trust in science and scientists, *Public Opinion Quarterly*, 83(4), 817–836.

References

Kreko, P. 2020. Countering conspiracy theories and misinformation. In *Routledge Handbook of Conspiracy Theories*, Eds M. Butter and P. Knight, London, Routledge.

Larson, H.J. 2020. Blocking information on COVID-19 can fuel the spread of misinformation, *Nature*, 580, 306.

Landrum, A.R. and Olshansky, A. 2019. The role of conspiracy mentality in denial of science and susceptibility to viral deception about science, *Politics and the Life Sciences*, 38(2), 193–209.

Lavorgna, A. 2020. *Cybercrimes: Critical Issues in a Global Context*, London, Red Globe Press.

Lavorgna, A. 2021a. Looking and crime and deviancy in cyberspace through the social harm lens. In *Handbook of Social Harm*, Eds P.S. Leighton, T. Wyatt and P. Davies, London, Palgrave.

Lavorgna, A. 2021b. Epistemologies of cyberspace: notes for interdisciplinary research. In *Researching Cybercrimes: Methodologies, Ethics and Critical Approaches*, Eds A. Lavorgna and T.J. Holt, London, Palgrave.

Lavorgna, A. and Bishop, F. 2019. Framing of CAM-adjacent health scams in the UK media: an interdisciplinary perspective. In *Medical Misinformation and Social Harm in Non-Science-Based Health Practices: A Multidisciplinary Perspective*, Eds A. Lavorgna and A. Di Ronco, London, Routledge.

Lavorgna, A. and Carr, L. 2021. Tweets and quacks: network and content analyses of providers of non-science-based anti-cancer treatments and their supporters on Twitter, Sage Open.

Lavorgna, A., Carr, L. and Kingdon, A. 2021. To wear or not to wear? Unpacking the #NoMask discourses and conversations on Twitter.

Lavorgna, A. and Di Ronco, A. 2017. Fraud victims or unwary accomplices? An exploratory study of online communities supporting quack medicine. In *The Many Faces of Crime for Profit and Ways of Tackling It*, Eds P.C. van Duyne, J. Harvey, G.A. Antonopoulos and K. von Lampe, Oisterwijk, Wolf Legal Publishers.

Lavorgna, A. and Di Ronco, A. 2018. Media representations of complementary and alternative medicine in the Italian press: a criminological perspective, *European Journal of Criminology*, 15(4), 421–441.

Lavorgna, A. and Di Ronco, A. 2019. Introduction. In *Medical Misinformation and Social Harm in Non-Science-Based Health Practices: A Multidisciplinary Perspective*, Eds A. Lavorgna and A. Di Ronco, London, Routledge.

Lavorgna, A. and Holt, T. J. Eds 2021. *Researching Cybercrimes: Methodologies, Ethics and Critical Approaches*, London, Palgrave.

Lavorgna, A. and Horsburgh, H. 2019. Towards a better criminological understanding of harmful alternative health practices: a provider typology. In *Medical Misinformation and Social Harm in Non-Science-Based Health Practices: A Multidisciplinary Perspective*, Eds A. Lavorgna and A. Di Ronco, London, Routledge.

Lavorgna, A. and Myles, H. 2021. Science denial and medical misinformation in pandemic times: a psycho-criminological analysis, *European Journal of Criminology* (online first).

Lavorgna, A. and Sugiura, L. 2019. Caught in a lie: the rise and fall of a respectable deviant, *Deviant Behaviour*, 40(9), 1043–1056.

Lavorgna, A. and Sugiura, L. 2020. Direct contacts with potential interviewees when carrying out online ethnography on controversial and polarized topics: a loophole in ethics guidelines, *International Journal of Social Research Methodology* (online first).

Leone, M., Madisson, M.L. and Ventsel, A. 2020. Semiotic approaches to conspiracy theories. In *Routledge Handbook of Conspiracy Theories*, Eds M. Butter and P. Knight, London, Routledge.

Lerner, I.J. 1984. The whys of cancer quackery, *Cancer*, 53, 815–819.

Lettera Aperta. 2020. *Tracciamento dei contatti e democrazia: Lettera aperta ai decisori*. Nexa center for Internet & Society. Available at: https://nexa.polito.it/lettera-aperta-app-COVID19?fbclid=IwAR2FdgZ9zTCwTa6GPCpR-k1ReBgwd6AOp6UWpviz1o1JZr92qT7MUzQvucE

Licoppe, C. and Inada, Y. 2012. "Timid encounters": A case study in the use of proximity-based mobile technologies. In *Proceedings of the SIGCHI Conference on Human Factors in Computing Systems*, Austin, Texas.

Loseke, D.R. 2007. The study of identity as cultural, institutional, organizational, and personal narratives: theoretical and empirical integrations, *The Sociological Quarterly*, 48(4), 661–688.

Mackey, T.K. and Liang, B.A. 2017. Health advertising in the digital age. Future trends and challenges. In *Digital Advertising. Theory and Research*, Eds S. Rodgers and E. Thorson, London, Routledge.

Mackie, D.M., Devos, T. and Smith, E.R. 2000. Intergroup emotions: explaining offensive action tendencies in an intergroup context, *Journal of Personality and Social Psychology*, 79(4), 602–616.

Mandoki, K. 2016. *Everyday Aesthetics: Prosaics, the Play of Culture and Social Identities*. New York, NY, Routledge.

Maratea, R.J. and Kavanaugh, P.R. 2012. Deviant identity in online contexts: new directives in the study of a classic concept, *Sociology Compass*, 6(2), 102–112.

Marino, G. and Serani, D. 2020. Dal #iorestoacasa alla ripartenza: gli utenti italiani di internet e l'informazione nelle due fasi dell'emergenza. I dati longitudinali del progetto I-POLHYS, *Problemi dell'informazione*, 3, 513–518.

Martin, H. and Debons, J. 2015. CAM and conventional medicine in Switzerland. Dovided in theory, united in practice. In *Routledge Handbook of Complementary and Alternative Medicine. Perspectives from Social Science and Law*, Eds N.K. Gale and J.V. McHale, London, Routledge.

Martin, R. and Johnson, L. Eds 2001. *Law and the Public Dimension of Health*, London, Routledge.

Martin, S. 2017. Word-of-mouth in the health care sector: a literature analysis of the current state of research and future perspectives, *International Review on Public and Nonprofit Marketing*, 14, 35–56.

Martinelli, A. 2018. Populism and Nationalism. The (peculiar) case of Italy. In *When Populism Meets Nationalism. Reflections on Parties in Power*, Ed. A. Martinelli, Milano, ISPI.

Martiny, S.E. and Rubin, M. 2016. Towards a clearer understanding of social identity theory's self-esteem hypothesis. In *Understanding Peace and Conflict through Social Identity Theory*, Eds S. McKeown, R. Haji and N. Ferguson, Cham, Springer.

Maruna, S. 2010. Mixed method research in criminology: why not go both ways?, In *Handbook of Quantitative Criminology*, Eds A. Piquero and D. Weisburd, New York, NY, Springer.

Mason, K.A., Willen, S.S., Holmes, S.M., Herd, D.A., Nichter, M., Castaneda, H. and Hansen, H. 2020. Critical analysis of challenges and opportunities for medical anthropology. *Population Health Management* (online first).

Massa, E. 2019. "Don't trust the experts!": Analysing the use of populist rhetoric in the anti-vaxxers discourse in Italy. In *Medical Misinformation and Social Harm in Non-Science-Based Health Practices: A Multidisciplinary Perspective*, Eds A. Lavorgna and A. Di Ronco, London: Routledge.

Matza, D. 1964. *Delinquency and Drift*, New York, NY, Wiley.

Matza, D. 1969. *Becoming Deviant*, Englewood Cliffs, NJ, Prentice Hall.

Matza, D. and Sykes, G. 1961. Juvenile delinquency and subterranean values, *American Sociological Review*, 26, 712–719.

McCoy, S. and Major, B. 2003. Group identification moderates emotional responses to perceived prejudice, *Personality and Social Psychology Bulletin*, 29(8), 1005–1017.

McDonald, D.W. 2007. Visual conversation styles in Web communities. In *40th Annual Hawaii International Conference on System Sciences (HICSS'07)*, pp. 76–76, Waikoloa, HI.

McHale, J.V. 2015. Legal frameworks, professional regulation and CAM practice in England. Is CAM "the special one"? In *Routledge Handbook of Complementary and Alternative Medicine. Perspectives from Social Science and Law*, Eds N.K. Gale and J.V. McHale, London, Routledge.

McManus, S., D'Ardenne, J. and Wessely, S. 2020. Covid conspiracies: misleading evidence can be more damaging than no evidence at all, *Psychological Medicine*, 1–2. doi:10.1017/S0033291720002184

Mede, N.G. and Schafer, M.S. 2020. Science-related populism: conceptualizing populist demands toward science, *Public Understanding of Science* (online first).

Metin, D., Cakiroglu, J. and Leblebicioglu, G. 2020. Perceptions of eighth graders concerning the aim, effectiveness, and scientific basis of pseudoscience: the case of crystal healing, *Research in Science Education*, 50, 175–202.

Mirable, P. and Horne, Z. 2019. Explanatory virtues and belief in conspiracy theories, *PsyArXiv*, May 15. doi:10.31234/osf.io/5cu2g

Muncie, J. 2000. Decriminalizing criminology. In *Rethinking Social Policy*, Eds G. Lewis, S. Gerwitz and J. Clarke, London, Sage.

NCSC. 2020. *Cyber Experts Step In as Criminals Seek to Exploit Coronavirus Fears*. Available at: https://www.ncsc.gov.uk/news/cyber-experts-step-criminals-exploit-coronavirus

Nerlich, B. and McLeod, C. 2016. The dilemma of raising awareness "responsibly", *EMBO Reports Science & Society*, 17, 481–485.

O'Connor, C. and Weatherall, J.O. 2019. *The Misinformation Age*, New Haven, CT, Yale University Press.

References

O'Hara, K. and Hall, W. 2018. *Four Internets: The Geopolitics of Internet Governance*, Waterloo, The Centre for International Governance Innovation.

O'Reilly, K. 2005. *Ethnographic Methods*, London, Routledge.

Offit, P. 2013. *Killing Us Softly: The Sense and Nonsense of Alternative Medicine*, London, HarperCollins.

Oswald, S. 2016. Conspiracy and bias: argumentative features and persuasiveness of conspiracy theories, *OSSA Conference Archive*, 168, 1–16.

Pemberton, S. 2004. A theory of moral indifference: Understanding the production of harm by capitalist society. In *Beyond Criminology. Taking Harm Seriously*, Eds P. Hillyard, C. Pantazis, S. Tombs and D. Gordon, London, Pluto Press.

Pemberton, S. 2007. Social harm future(s): exploring the potential of the social harm approach, *Crime Law & Social Change*, 48(1–2), 27–41.

Pemberton, S. 2016. *Harmful Societies: Understanding Social Harm*, Bristol, Policy Press.

Peršak, N. 2007. *Criminalising Harmful Conduct: The Harm Principle, Its Limits and Continental Counterparts*, New York, NY, Springer.

Peruzzi, A., Zollo, F., Schmidt, A.L. and Quattrociocchi, W. 2019. From confirmation bias to echo-chambers: a data-driven approach, *Sociologia e Politiche Sociali*, 3, 47–74.

Peters, H.P. 2014. Scientists as public experts. Expectations and responsibilities. In *Routledge Handbook of Public Communication of Science and Technology*, Eds M. Bucchi and B. Trench, London, Routledge.

Pierre, J.M. 2020. Mistrust and misinformation: a two-component, socio-epistemic model of belief in conspiracy theories, *Journal of Social and Political Psychology*, 8(2), 617–641.

Pink, S., Horst, H., Postill, J., Hjorth, L., Lewis, T. and Tacchi, J. 2016. *Digital Ethnography: Principles and Practice*, London, Sage.

Pisano, G.P., Sadun, R. and Zanini, M. 2020. Lessons from Italy's response to coronavirus, *Harvard Business Review*, March 27. Available at: https://hbr.org/2020/03/lessons-from-italys-response-to-coronavirus

Pless, I.B. 2003. Expanding the precautionary principle, *Injury Prevention*, 9, 1–2.

Poland, G.A. and Jacobson, R.M. 2011. The age-old struggle against the antivaccinationists, *The New England Journal of Medicine*, 364, 97–99.

Popham, J. 2018. Microdeviation: observations on the significance of lesser harms in shaping the nature of cyberspace, *Deviant Behaviour*, 39(2), 159–169.

Popper, K.R. 1972. *Conjectures and Refutations*, 4th ed., London, Routledge.

Porter, C.E. 2004. A typology of virtual communities: a multi-disciplinary foundation for future research, *Journal of Computer-Mediated Communication*, 10(1), JCMC1011.

Postil, J. 2014. A critical history of Internet activism and social protest in Malaysia, 1998–2011, *Asiascape: Digital Asia Journal*, 1(2), 78–103.

Postill, J. and Pink, S. 2012. Social media ethnography: the digital researcher in a messy web, *Media International Australia*, 145, 123–134.

Powell, A. and Henry, N. 2017. *Sexual Violence in a Digital Age*, London, Palgrave Macmillan.

Powell, A., Stratton, G. and Cameron, R. 2018. *Digital Criminology*, New York, NY, Routledge.

Prot, S. and Anderson, C. A. (2019). Science denial. Psychological processes underlying denial of science-based medical practices. In *Medical Misinformation and Social Harm in Non-Science-Based Health Practices. A Multidisciplinary Perspective*, Eds A. Lavorgna and A. Di Ronco, London, Routledge.

Quinn, K., Epstein, D. and Moon, B. 2019. We care about different things: non-elite conceptualizations of social media privacy, *Social Media + Society*, 5(3), 1–14.

Raban, J. 1974. *Soft City*, London, Hamilton.

Ratzan, S.C., Bloom, B.R., El-Mohandes, A., Fielding, J., Gostin, L.O., Hodge, J.G., Hotez, P., Kurth, A., Larson, H.J., Nurse, J., Omer, S.A., Orenstein, W.A., Salmon, D. and Rabin, K. 2019. The Salzburg statement on vaccination acceptance, *Journal of Health Communication*, 24(5), 581–583.

Remain, J.H. 1979. *The Rich Get Richer and the Poor Get Prison*, London, Wiley.

Richter, E.D., Laster, R. and Soskolne, C. 2005. The precautionary principle, epidemiology and the ethics of delay, *Human and Ecological Risk Assessment: An International Journal*, 11(1), 17–27.

Rimke, H.M. 2000. Governing citizens through self-help literature, *Cultural Studies*, 14(1), 61–78.

Ritzer, G. and Jurgenson, N. 2010. Production, consumption, presumption: the nature of capitalism in the age of the digital "prosumer", *Journal of Consumer Culture*, 10(1), 13–36.

Rojek, C. 2017. The case of Belle Gibson, social media, and what it means for understanding leisure under digital praxis, *Annals of Leisure Research*, 20(5), 524–528.

Rutjens, B.T. and van der Lee, R. 2020. Spiritual scepticism? Heterogeneous science scepticism in the Netherlands, *Public Understanding of Science* (online first).

Sacks, H. 1992. *Lectures on Conversation*, Vols. 1 and 2, Oxford, Blackwell.

Saks, M. 2015. Power and professionalisation in CAM. A sociological approach. In *Routledge Handbook of Complementary and Alternative Medicine. Perspectives from Social Science and Law*, Eds N.K. Gale and J.V. McHale, London, Routledge.

Shaluf, I.M., Ahmadun, F. and Mat Said, A. 2003. A review of disaster and crisis *Disaster Prevention and Management*, 12(1), 24–32.

Schmidt, A. and Wiegand, M. 2017. A survey in hate speech detection using natural language processing. In *Proceedings of the Workshop AFNLP SIG SocialNLP*.

Schmidt, A., Zollo, F., Scala, A., Betsch, C. and Quattrociocchi, W. 2018. Polarization of the vaccination debate on Facebook, *Vaccine*, 36(25), 3606–3612.

Schütze, F. 1983. Biographieforschung und narratives interview, *Neue Praxis*, 13(3), 283–293.

Sharon, A.J. and Baram-Tsabari, A. 2020. The experts' perspective of "ask-an-expert": An interview-based study of online nutrition and vaccination outreach, *Public Understanding of Science*, 29(3), 252–269.

Sherman, D.K. and Cohen, J.L. 2006. The psychology of self-defense: self-affirmation theory. In *Advances in Experimental Social Psychology*, Ed. M.P. Zanna, Vol. 38, San Diego: Academic Press.

Siani, A. 2019. Measles outbreaks in Italy: a paradigm of the re-emergence of vaccine-preventable diseases in developed countries, *Preventive Medicine*, 121, 99–104.

Simester, A.P. and Von Hirsch, A. 2011. *Crimes, Harms, and Wrongs: On the Principles of Criminalisation*, Oxford, Hart Publishing.

Smart, P., Ming-chin, M., O'Hara, K., Carr, L. and Hall, W. 2019. *Geopolitical Drivers of Personal Data: The Four Horsemen of the Datapocalypse*, Southampton, University of Southampton.

Smith, E.R., Seger, C.R. and Mackie, D.M. 2007. Can emotions be truly group level? Evidence regarding four conceptual criteria, *Journal of Personality and Social Psychology*, 93(3), 431–446.

Social Data Lab. 2019. Lab online guide to social media research ethics. Available at: http://socialdatalab.net/ethics-resources

Sommers, C. 1994. *Who Stole Feminism? How Women Have Betrayed Women*, New York, NY, Simon & Schuster.

Speck, P., Higginson, I. and Addington-Hall, J. 2004. Spiritual needs in health care, *BMJ*, 329, 123–124.

Stano, S. 2020. The internet and the spread of conspiracy content. In *Routledge Handbook of Conspiracy Theories*, Eds M. Butter and P. Knight, London, Routledge.

Stanovich, K.E., West, R.F. and Toplak, M.E. 2013. Myside bias, rational thinking, and intelligence, *Current Directions in Psychological Science*, 22, 259–264.

Stephan, W.G., Boniecki, K.A., Ybarra, O., Bettencourt, A., Ervin, K.S., Jackson, L.A., McNatt, P. and Renfro, L. 2002. The role of threats in the racial attitudes of Blacks and Whites, *Personality and Social Psychology Bulletin*, 28, 1242–1254.

Sugiura, L. 2018. *Respectable Deviance and Online Medicine Purchasing: Opportunities and Risks for Consumers*, Basingstoke, Palgrave Pivot.

Sykes, G. and Matza, D. 1957. Techniques of neutralization: a history of delinquency, *American Sociological Review*, 22, 664–670.

Szafranski, R. 1995. A theory of information warfare: preparing for 2020, *Airpower Journal*, 9(1), 56–65.

Tanyi, R.A. 2002. Towards clarification of the meaning of spirituality, *Journal of Advanced Nursing*, 39, 500–509.

Thalmann, K. 2019. *The Stigmatization of Conspiracy Theory since the 1950s*, London, Routledge.

References

The Guardian. 2020a. *As Coronavirus Spreads, I Am Terrified that Fear and Greed Could Cost My Son His Life*, March 9. Available at: https://www.theguardian.com/commentisfree/2020/mar/10/as-coronavirus-spreads-i-am-terrified-that-australias-fear-and-greed-could-cost-my-son-his-life

The Guardian. 2020b. *Vital Drug for People with Lupus Running Out After Unproven COVID-19 Link*, March 27. Available at: https://www.theguardian.com/world/2020/mar/27/vital-drug-people-lupus-coronavirus-covid-19-link-hydroxychloroquine

Thompson, W.E. and Gibbs, J.C. 2017. *Deviance and Deviants. A Sociological Approach*, Chichester, Wiley.

Tinati, R., Halford, S., Carr, L. and Pope, C. 2012. Mixing methods and theory to explore web activity. In *Proceedings of the 2012 ACM Conference on Web Science*, pp. 308–316. Evanston, Illinois.

Tsay-Vogel, M., Shanahan, J. and Signorielli, N. 2018. Social media cultivating perceptions of privacy: a 5-year analysis of privacy attitudes and self-disclosure behaviors among Facebook users, *New Media & Society*, 20(1), 141–161.

Urquiza-Haas, N. and Cloatre, E. 2019. Traditional herbal medicine and the challenges of pharmacovigilance. In *Medical Misinformation and Social Harm in Non-Science-Based Health Practices: A Multidisciplinary Perspective*, Eds A. Lavorgna and A. Di Ronco, London, Routledge.

Vineis, P. 2005. Scientific basis for the precautionary principle, *Toxicology and Applied Pharmacology*, 207(2), 658–662.

Virtanen, S.M. 2017. Fear of cybercrime in Europe: examining the effects of victimization and vulnerabilities, *Psychiatry, Psychology and Law*, 24(3), 323–338.

Wall, D.S. 2007. *Cybercrime: The Transformation of Crime in the Information Age*, Cambridge, Polity.

Webber, C. and Yip, M. 2013. Drifting on and off-line. Humanising the cyber criminal. In *New Directions in Crime and Delinquency*, Eds S. Winlow and R. Atkinson, London, Routledge.

Weeks, L.C. and Strudsholm, T. 2008. A scoping review of research on complementary and alternative medicine (CAM) and the mass media: looking back, moving forward, *BMC Complementary and Alternative Medicine*, 8(43), 1–9.

WHO. 2020. *Shortage of Personal Protective Equipment Endangering Health Workers Worldwide*, March 3. Available at: https://www.who.int/news-room/detail/03-03-2020-shortage-of-personal-protective-equipment-endangering-health-workers-worldwide

Williams, M.L., Burnap, P. and Sloan, L. 2017. Towards an ethical framework for publishing Twitter data in social research: taking into account users' views, online context and algorithmic estimation, *Sociology*, 51(6), 1149–1168.

Wired. 2020. Hackers Are Targeting Hospitals Crippled by Coronavirus, March 22. Available at: https://www.wired.co.uk/article/coronavirus-hackers-cybercrime-phishing

Wardle, C. and Derakhshan, H. 2017. *Information Disorder: Toward an Interdisciplinary Framework for Research and Policy Making*, Strasbourg, Council of Europe.

Yar, M. 2014. *Crime, Deviance and Doping: Fallen Sports Star, Autobiography and the Management of Stigma*, Basingstoke, Palgrave Macmillan.

Young, J. 1999. Cannibalism and bulimia: patterns of social control in late modernity, *Theoretical Criminology*, 3(4), 387–407.

Young, J. 2003. Merton with energy, Katz with structure. The sociology of vindictiveness and the criminology of transgression, *Theoretical Criminology*, 7(3), 389–414.

Zarocostas, J. 2020. How to fight an infodemic, *The Lancet*, 395(102225), P676.

Zedner, L. 2007. Pre-crime and post-criminology, *Theoretical Criminology*, 11(2), 261–281.

Zhu, Y., Guan, M. and Donovan, E. 2020. Elaborating cancer opinion leaders' communication behaviours within online health communities: network and content analyses, *Social Media + Society*, 6(2). https://doi.org/10.1177/2056305120909473

Zimmer, M. and Kinder-Kurlanda, K. Eds 2017. *Research Ethics for the Social Age. New Challenges, Cases, and Contexts*, New York, NY, Peter Lang.

Zinn, J. 2008. Heading into the unknown: everyday strategies for managing risk and uncertainty, *Health, Risks and Society*, 10(5), 439–450.

INDEX

Academia, 4
Academic, 11, 34, 40
   imaginaries, 45
   jurisdiction, 57
Activist, 4, 57
Actor, 27, 51, 63
Agency, 12, 25, 39, 44, 53–55, 60
Alternative, 4–6, 8, 18, 29–31, 35, 38, 40, 46, 61, 65
Anonymity, 19
Anthropology, 17
Antivax, 6, 51
   beliefs, 54
   clusters, 6
   communicative strategies in, 65
Architectural change, 63
Argumentation, 41
Attachment, 28
Autism, 6
Automatic, 7, 31

Belief, 7, 22, 29, 34
   antivax, 54
   conspiracy, 39–40, 41, 43, 55, 60, 65
   health-related beliefs, 60
   neutralizing, 24
   perseverance, 41
   philosophical, 19
   spiritual, 55
Belonging, 17, 28, 34, 43
   of CAMs, 62
   outgroup hostility and ingroup, 46, 49
Big data, 7, 15, 50
   digital positivism on, 15

Body, 4, 46, 53, 55, 57
Bulimic society, 26, 58
Business as usual, 13, 33

CAM, 4
   community, 37
   intervention and monitoring, 63
   researchers, 62
Catalysis event, 28, 32–33
Celebrity, 34, 63
Children, 30, 36, 53, 54
China, 1, 51
Choice, 24, 30, 50, 53, 61
Collective, 5, 11, 25, 52
   moral agents, 61
   moral responsibility, 60–61
Community, 28, 30, 33, 37, 41, 46, 49, 54, 60
Conspiracy, 6, 31, 51, 66
   beliefs, 39, 42
   conspiracy-led narratives, 38
Conspiratorial thinking, 38–39, 41
Contagion, 1, 3, 48
Context, 5
   of COVID-19, 21
   of crime and deviancy, 13
   of crossdisciplinarity, 57–59
   cultural and discursive, 7
   culture, 25
   exploratory psycho-criminological analysis, 18
   of health-related information, 9–10
   information, 41
   of interdisciplinary analyses, 17
   medical, 63

medical misinformation, 15
of medical misinformation, 61
of pandemic, 14, 32, 53
of public health, 60
of social networks, 44
of systemically underfunded education sector, 32
of technology-facilitated social harms, 2, 44, 55, 57, 63
of vaccination, 66
Control, 10, 67
  compensatory sense of, 39
  crime, 25
  of information, 26
  institutional, 54
  sense of, 53
  social, 51
  social, 54, 65
Convergent technologies, 25, 32, 44, 60
Conversation, 3, 7, 18, 20–21, 28, 49, 60, 63
Coronavirus, 1, 11, 30, 36, 48, 57
Counter-culture, 39
Counterinformation, 3, 14, 50–51
COVID-19, 1, 12–13, 17–18, 21, 31, 38, 48, 54, 63
Covidiot, 47–48
Crime, 2, 9, 54
  crime control industry, 10
  during pandemic, 13
  prevention and reduction, 25
Criminology, 4, 9, 15, 22, 25
Crisis, 2, 12, 50, 53, 58
Critical care, 1
Crossdisciplinarity, 57
Culpability, 10
Cultural, 4, 5
  cognition affects, 66
  contexts, 7
  criminology, 22, 25–26
  spaces, 25
  values, 66
Culture, 10, 25, 38–39, 47, 50

Cybersanctioning, 65
Cyberspace, 4, 9, 10, 14, 24, 53, 59, 64

Data science, 4, 6
Dataveillance, 38
Death, 1, 54, 65
Debunker, 4, 33, 64
Debunking, 8, 65, 67
Decree, 1
Defensiveness, 47
Denial, 17, 45, 52, 66
Deprivation, 39, 51, 58
Determinism, 24, 58
Deviance, 2, 9–10, 16, 22–23, 25
Deviant, 2, 16, 22–23, 25
Digital, 9, 15, 18, 20, 28, 44, 50, 59
Disease, 6, 31, 53, 57
Displacement, 67
Displacing, 14, 33, 54
Distancing, 14, 33–34, 54
Doctor, 29, 32–34, 37, 44, 62, 64
Doubt, 5, 8, 30, 44
Drift, 23, 32, 50, 58, 60
Dual city, 16
Duration, 49, 60

Echo chamber, 7, 50
Education, 29, 32, 37, 53
Effective, 4, 9, 13, 25, 62, 66, 67
Elite, 38, 40, 45–46
Emergency, 33, 38, 56
Emotion, 66
Empowerment, 5, 53, 55
Epistemic mistrust, 38, 40
Epistemology, 15, 40
Establishment, 5, 33, 31, 34, 37
Ethic, 19, 21, 26, 37, 44
Ethnography, 18, 22, 30, 36, 51, 55, 57
Europe, 1
European, 2, 42, 46, 51–52
Event, 9–10, 32–33, 37, 54
Exceptionalism, 13

Existentialism, 19
Expert, 6, 33, 40, 43–44, 54, 59, 66
Expertise, 5, 44, 59, 64
Exposure, 21–23, 56, 58, 60

Facebook, 18, 29, 30–31
Fact-checking, 65
Fake, 3–4, 35, 44–45
Fear, 2, 8, 49, 56, 64–65
Feminism, 53
Filter bubble, 50
Filtering, 6–7
Forum, 19
Frame, 27, 43–44, 60
Framing, 1, 21
Fraud, 4–6, 8, 10, 12, 45
Freedom, 23, 29, 52, 56, 58
Frequency, 34, 49, 60
Fringe, 29, 39, 46, 65

Galileo, 46
Gender, 53
Government, 31, 38, 46, 54

Harassment, 21
Harm, 1, 5, 9, 22, 2
Harmful, 8, 11, 25, 58, 62
Health, 1, 4, 13, 17, 28, 31, 37, 41, 47, 53, 56–57, 62, 66
 health-related beliefs, 60
 individual moral responsibility in, 61
Healthcare, 1, 4, 5, 12–13
Help, 13–14, 16, 30, 36, 40, 58
Heretics, 46
Hope, 4, 29, 36, 38, 64
Hospital, 12, 30, 47
Hospitalization, 1, 49
Hostility, 46
Hygiene theatre, 32

Identity, 22, 25, 27, 34, 42–43, 46, 49, 51, 58
Ideology, 52, 66

Illness, 5, 55
Image, 19–20, 43, 48, 55, 64
Immigration, 51
Immuni, 56
Impact, 1–2, 4, 8, 10, 13, 19, 41, 66
Impression, 6, 27
Incentive, 4, 65
Individual, 2, 5, 6, 9, 12, 15, 20, 24, 33, 39, 46, 50, 53, 55, 66
Infodemic, 3
Information pollution, 2–3, 9, 12–13, 16, 59
Ingroup, 25, 39, 48, 49
Injustice, 23, 26, 39–40
Intensity, 49, 60
Intensive care, 1, 3, 47
Interviews, 17, 21, 42, 56
Intragroup, 41, 43
Involvement, 23, 28–29, 34
Irrational, 66
Italy, 1–2, 51–52, 54, 62, 64

Knowledge, 2–5, 11, 21, 40–42, 45, 59, 65

Late modernity, 5, 26, 64
Legal, 9, 11, 25, 54
Legitimacy, 5, 10, 23, 33, 35, 62
LGBTQ, 53
Libertarian, 52–53, 60
Liberty, 39, 66
Lifestyle, 3, 14, 18, 31, 53
Lockdown, 2, 13, 17, 47, 52, 54
Lombardia, 13, 17, 32, 49, 52, 54

Mala in se, 2
Mask, 8, 13, 33, 42, 51, 24
Media, 39, 41–42, 51, 55, 56, 59, 61–64
Medicine, 4, 12, 35, 61
Meme, 19, 20, 47–48
Mental health, 2
Methodology, 25

Micro-deviation, 10
Misinformation, 3, 5, 7, 9, 13, 22, 44, 57, 60–61
Mistrust, 38, 40, 51, 65
Moral, 11, 30, 35, 52, 61
Morality, 44
Motivation, 7, 20, 27, 31, 36
Movement, 47, 51, 54
Music, 48

Narrative, 44, 60, 64
Natural Language Processing 7
Negligence, 10, 35
Net neutrality, 60
Network, 2, 28, 34, 43, 58, 61
Normalization, 16
Nurse, 30, 35

Official, 21, 33, 37, 41–42, 45, 54
Offline, 16, 31–32, 34, 58
Online intermediaries, 7, 61, 63, 67
Outbreak, 1–2, 6, 13, 18
Outgroup, 39, 40, 46, 54
Outsider, 40, 46, 54

Pandemic, 1–3, 30, 55, 57, 61, 64
Parent, 6, 32
Parrhesia, 41
Paternal internet, 60
Patient, 5, 31, 35
PayPal, 36
Pedagogical philosophies, 53
Permits, 54
Pharma, 35
Placebo, 5, 22
Platform, 4, 42, 44, 56, 63
Polarization, 67
Polarized logic, 6, 13, 22, 39
Policymaking, 64
Political homogeneity, 3, 7, 16, 19, 39, 51
Politics, 19, 25, 50–51
Populism, 4, 45
Positivism, 15

Power, 22, 35, 39, 41, 44, 48, 56
Pragmatism, 58
Precautionary principle, 13
Predatory, 44–45
Presentation, 3, 27, 43
Prevention, 25, 66–67
Preventive measures, 29, 31, 48, 51, 52, 54, 62
Primrose, 54
Privacy, 55–56
Private companies, 5, 12, 22, 42, 50, 56, 61
Professional, 14, 29, 37, 62, 64
Profit, 36
Propagator, 17, 27
Protective behaviors, 8, 33
Provider, 27, 31, 66
Pseudoscience, 4, 38
Psychology, 4, 17
Public, 1, 8, 18, 29, 37, 49, 60–61, 64, 66
Public health, 1, 13, 60, 63, 66
Publication, 42, 44–45, 56, 60
Published, 3, 18, 20, 36

Qanon, 38
Quack, 4, 10, 37
Qualitative analyses, 15–16, 25, 50, 58
Quality, 34, 60
Quarantine, 1

Radical right, 51
Rational calculation, 17, 40, 44, 65
Reactance, 52
Reason, 3, 7, 18, 35, 62, 64, 66
Receiver, 3, 28–29, 32, 45, 59
Regulation, 10, 27, 62
Regulatory frameworks, 7, 10, 12, 61–63
Religion, 55
Religious identification, 16, 19, 52–53
Reputable, 34, 45
Reputation, 34, 36

Index

Researcher, 44, 56, 64
Responsibility, 8, 11, 30, 35, 39, 53, 61–63
Right to try, 29
Risk, 10, 16–17, 26, 48, 58, 66

Safe, 4, 21, 34, 39
Safety, 6, 8–9, 12, 33, 37
School, 32–33, 53
Science, 4, 6, 16–17, 37, 40, 45–46, 55, 64, 66
Science communication, 17, 64
Scientific establishment, 45–46, 52, 64, 66
Scientist, 33, 44, 64
Scientocracy, 45
Self, 5, 19, 43, 53, 55
Self-help, 5
Situational contexts, 23, 32–33, 50, 61
Skeptic, 33, 41, 64
Social harms, 1, 11, 14, 16, 57, 61, 64
Social media, 4–5, 8, 16, 19, 21, 29, 33, 42, 51, 59, 67
Social sciences, 20, 57–58
Socialization, 16–17, 24, 43, 58, 60
Socio-technical approach, 59
Sociology, 4, 25
Spiritual, 14, 55, 65
Spirituality, 55
State, 12, 29, 36, 38, 53
Status, 21, 29, 43, 46, 62, 64–65
Stereotype, 40, 60, 39, 57, 65
Stigmatization, 39, 57, 65
Storytelling, 20, 27, 41, 44
Subcultural theories, 23, 28
Subculture, 24–25, 43
Success, 7, 22, 39, 54, 59–60
Support, 5, 13, 25, 27, 31, 49, 55

Supporter, 20, 30–31–33, 59, 64
Symbol, 49, 54

Technical intervention, 50, 59
Technological sophistication, 7, 10, 16
Technology, 2, 18, 22, 38, 64
Telegram, 32, 50
Television, 32, 44, 64
Test, 12
Testing, 12–13, 56
Training, 37, 44
Transgression, 25, 30, 46
Trust, 5, 8, 21, 63, 66
Truth, 41–42, 49, 56, 64
Twitter, 33

Uncertainty, 17
United States, 12–13, 51, 53
Us *vs.* them narrative, 24, 36, 39, 46, 52, 64
Utilizer, 27–29

Vaccination, 6, 32, 38, 54, 61
Vaccine, 12, 29, 38, 54, 65
Validation, 35–36
Victim, 9, 14, 29, 30, 35, 40
Video, 20, 29, 42, 48, 55
Vulnerability, 31, 33, 57, 63
Vulnerable victims, 2, 9, 13, 35, 54

Wave, 2, 17, 30, 49
Website, 7–8, 18–19, 31, 36
Wellbeing, 4, 22, 55
Wellness, 31, 36, 51
WhatsApp, 32, 50
World Health Organization (WHO), 1

YouTube, 42

Printed in the United States
by Baker & Taylor Publisher Services